Sustainable Living and Eco-Friendly Tips

Practical Tips for Adopting a Greener Lifestyle

Elo Marc

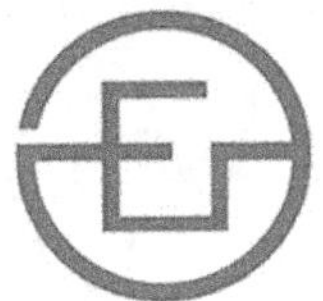

Introduction

In a world where environmental concerns are more pressing than ever, adopting a sustainable and eco-friendly lifestyle can significantly impact the planet's health. This book aims to provide practical tips and insights to help you lead a greener life, from reducing waste to incorporating sustainable habits and eco-friendly products. By making small, intentional changes in your everyday life, you can contribute to a healthier planet.

Elo Marc

Chapter 1
Understanding Sustainability and Its Importance

Sustainability is a concept that has become central to the way we live, work, and interact with the world. This chapter will explore what sustainability means, why it is so crucial for both the environment and society, and how adopting sustainable practices can make a real difference.

Defining Sustainability: What Does It Mean to Live Sustainably?

At its core, sustainability refers to the ability to meet the needs of the present without compromising the ability of future generations to meet their own needs. It involves making choices that minimize negative impacts on the planet, society, and future generations while balancing economic and social development.

Living sustainably means making conscious decisions that preserve resources, reduce waste, and promote long-term ecological balance. It is a way of life that focuses on using resources in a manner that keeps ecosystems intact, supports economic stability, and fosters social equity.

Key aspects of sustainable living include:

• **Conserving Resources**: Using resources wisely and avoiding depletion.

• **Reducing Environmental Impact**: Minimizing pollution, waste, and carbon footprints.

• **Supporting Ethical Practices**: Encouraging businesses and communities to act responsibly.

• **Promoting Equity and Justice**: Ensuring that sustainability benefits all people, especially marginalized communities.

Why Sustainability Matters: The Environmental and Social Impacts of Unsustainable Practices

Unsustainable practices—such as overconsumption, pollution, deforestation, and the exploitation of resources—have led to many environmental and social problems. These issues affect not only the planet but also communities and economies worldwide.

Environmental Impacts:

• **Climate Change:** The burning of fossil fuels and industrial practices have significantly increased greenhouse gases in the atmosphere, causing global temperatures to rise and leading to extreme weather events.

• **Resource Depletion:** Overuse of nonrenewable resources, such as fossil fuels and minerals, is putting pressure on ecosystems and wildlife, reducing biodiversity.

• **Pollution:** Chemical pollution from agriculture, industries, and waste is contaminating water, air, and soil, affecting ecosystems and human health.

• **Deforestation and Habitat Loss:** The destruction of

forests for agriculture and urbanization leads to the loss of biodiversity and disrupts ecosystems.

Social Impacts:

• **Inequality:** Unsustainable economic practices can widen the gap between rich and poor, leading to greater social inequality and limiting access to resources for vulnerable populations.

• **Health Risks:** Pollution and exposure to hazardous chemicals lead to diseases and health problems, particularly in underserved communities.

• **Displacement and Conflict:** Resource scarcity can lead to conflicts, displacement, and migration, especially in regions heavily affected by environmental degradation.

Sustainability addresses these issues by advocating for practices that protect the planet, foster social well-being, and promote fairness and justice for all communities.

The Three Pillars of Sustainability: Environmental, Social, and Economic Sustainability

Sustainability is often described in terms of three interconnected pillars, each of which plays a vital role in creating a balanced, sustainable world. These pillars—**environmental**, **social**, and **economic** sustainability—are essential for achieving long-term sustainability.

1. Environmental Sustainability:

o This pillar focuses on preserving natural resources, reducing pollution, and maintaining biodiversity. It involves making choices that protect the planet's ecosystems, such as reducing carbon emissions, conserving water, and using renewable energy sources.

○ **Key principles**: conservation, biodiversity, waste reduction, pollution control, and renewable energy.

2. Social Sustainability:

○ Social sustainability is concerned with creating fair, equitable, and just communities. It involves ensuring that all individuals have access to basic needs such as clean air and water, education, healthcare, and a safe environment.

○ **Key principles**: equity, justice, community well-being, human rights, and access to opportunities for all people.

3. Economic Sustainability:

○ Economic sustainability focuses on creating a stable economy that provides long-term prosperity without depleting resources or causing social harm. It involves promoting sustainable business practices, creating green jobs, and fostering economic policies that encourage innovation and fair distribution of wealth.

○ **Key principles**: responsible economic growth, green jobs, fair trade, and sustainable business models.

When all three pillars work in harmony, we can achieve a truly sustainable world where the needs of people and the planet are met without sacrificing future generations' ability to thrive.

Your Role in Sustainability: How Individual Actions Contribute to Global Change

Every individual has the power to make a difference. While large-scale change requires policy shifts and collective action, the choices you make every day can have a significant impact on the environment and society. By adopting sustainable habits, you can contribute to global efforts to combat climate change, reduce waste, and create a more just and equitable world.

Ways to contribute as an individual:

• **Reduce, Reuse, Recycle**: Practice waste reduction at home and in the workplace. Buy less, repurpose old items, and recycle whenever possible.

• **Support Ethical Brands**: Choose products from companies that prioritize sustainability, fair wages, and ethical sourcing.

• **Conserve Resources**: Use water and energy efficiently by making simple changes, like turning off lights, fixing leaks, and using energy-efficient appliances.

• **Advocate for Change**: Support policies and organizations that promote sustainability, such as clean energy initiatives, waste reduction programs, and environmental conservation efforts.

• **Educate and Inspire Others**: Share your knowledge of sustainability with friends, family, and coworkers. Lead by example and inspire others to adopt eco-friendly habits.

By understanding the importance of sustainability, recognizing the interconnectedness of the environmental, social, and economic pillars, and embracing your personal role in driving change, you can contribute to a global movement toward a more sustainable future. Every action, no matter how small, counts toward creating a healthier, fairer, and more sustainable world for all.

To Keep In Mind: Sustainability is not just a buzzword—it is a necessary framework for ensuring the future health of our planet and its inhabitants. The choices we make today will determine the world we leave for future generations. By understanding sustainability and integrating it into our daily lives, we can be part of the solution to the global challenges we face.

Chapter 2
Reducing Waste in Your Daily Life

In today's world, waste has become a significant environmental challenge. From landfills overflowing with discarded items to the pollution caused by single-use plastics, the need to reduce waste has never been more urgent. In this chapter, we'll explore practical strategies for reducing waste in your daily life, focusing on the principles of the zero-waste movement, mindful consumption, upcycling, and waste-free kitchen tips.

The Zero-Waste Movement: What Is It, and How Can You Practice It?

The zero-waste movement is a lifestyle aimed at reducing the amount of waste we generate, ideally striving to send nothing to a landfill or incinerator. It is based on the principle that we should consume and dispose of resources in ways that minimize harm to the environment. This includes rethinking how we buy, use, and dispose of products and materials.

Key principles of zero waste:

• **Refuse**: Say no to unnecessary items, such as free promotional products, plastic bags, or excessive packaging.

• **Reduce**: Limit your consumption by purchasing fewer, higher-quality items that last longer.

• **Reuse**: Opt for items that can be reused instead of disposable ones, such as cloth bags, glass containers, and metal straws.

• **Recycle**: Make sure to recycle whenever possible, and educate yourself on local recycling programs to avoid contamination.

• **Rot**: Compost food scraps and yard waste to turn organic materials into valuable resources for your garden.

How to practice zero waste:

• **Start small**: Begin by focusing on one area of your life, such as reducing plastic waste, and gradually expand your efforts.

• **Switch to reusable products**: Replace single-use items like water bottles, coffee cups, and plastic cutlery with reusable versions made of stainless steel, glass, or bamboo.

• **Mind your packaging**: Choose products with minimal packaging or opt for bulk goods that allow you to use your own containers.

By incorporating these zero-waste practices into your daily routine, you'll reduce your environmental impact and help prevent waste from accumulating in landfills.

Mindful Consumption: Buying Less and Choosing Quality Over Quantity

One of the most effective ways to reduce waste is by practicing mindful consumption—being intentional about the items we buy and the resources we use. In a world where we're constantly bombarded with marketing messages encouraging us to buy more, it's easy to fall into the trap of overconsumption. Mindful consumption, however, encourages us to pause and make thoughtful decisions that benefit both us and the planet.

Tips for practicing mindful consumption:

• **Buy less, choose wisely**: Before purchasing, ask yourself whether the item is truly necessary, how often you'll use it, and whether it will add long-term value to your life. Opt for high-quality items that will last longer rather than cheap, disposable alternatives.

• **Research brands**: Choose products from companies that prioritize sustainability, ethical production, and environmentally friendly packaging. Look for certifications like Fair Trade, B Corp, or Energy Star.

• **Embrace minimalism**: Focus on owning only what you truly need and love. Decluttering your home and wardrobe not only reduces waste but can also help you live more intentionally.

• **Repair and repurpose**: Instead of discarding broken items, consider repairing them or repurposing them for another use. This can reduce the demand for new products and minimize waste.

By being mindful of what and how much we buy, we reduce the pressure on our environment, conserve natural resources, and avoid the waste associated with fast fashion and disposable goods.

Upcycling and Repurposing: Giving Items a Second Life

Upcycling and repurposing are powerful ways to reduce waste by turning unwanted or discarded items into something useful or beautiful again. Rather than sending things to the landfill, you can give them a second life and reduce the need for new resources.

What is upcycling?

• **Upcycling** involves transforming an item that would otherwise be thrown away into something more valuable or useful. This can range from turning old furniture into something new to creatively using everyday items in innovative ways.

How to upcycle and repurpose:

• **Furniture**: Old wooden furniture can be sanded down and refinished, or repurposed into new pieces such as shelves, tables, or even plant stands.

• **Clothing**: Turn worn-out clothes into new items like rags, patches, or even quilts. You can also transform old t-shirts into reusable tote bags.

• **Glass jars**: Instead of throwing out glass jars, use them for storage, as planters, or even turn them into decorative candle holders.

• **Old tires**: Tires can be upcycled into garden planters, swings, or outdoor furniture.

Upcycling not only helps keep waste out of landfills but also encourages creativity and resourcefulness. It's an opportunity to rethink the potential uses of everyday items and add a personal, sustainable touch to your home.

Waste-Free Kitchen Tips: Composting, Recycling, and Minimizing Food Waste

The kitchen is one of the biggest contributors to household waste, with food scraps, packaging, and disposable products accumulating quickly. However, by incorporating a few key habits, you can drastically reduce your kitchen waste and make your home more eco-friendly.

1. Composting: Composting is the process of turning food scraps and organic waste into nutrient-rich soil. Instead of throwing away vegetable peels, coffee grounds, and fruit scraps, you can compost them and use the resulting material to enrich your garden.

• **What to compost**: Fruit and vegetable scraps, coffee grounds, eggshells, grass clippings, and yard waste.

• **What not to compost**: Meat, dairy, oily foods, and pet waste.

2. Recycling: Recycling is another essential waste-reduction strategy. Make sure you separate recyclables from regular waste, following local recycling guidelines to avoid contamination.

• **Recyclable kitchen items**: Glass jars, aluminum cans, paper cartons, and plastic bottles (check local recycling programs for which plastics are accepted).

• **Avoid contamination**: Rinse recyclables to ensure they don't contaminate the recycling stream, which could render them unrecyclable.

3. Minimizing Food Waste: Food waste is a major problem worldwide, both from an environmental and social standpoint. There are many ways you can minimize food waste in the kitchen, including:

• **Plan meals**: Plan meals for the week to avoid overbuying ingredients that may spoil.

• **Use leftovers creatively**: Repurpose leftovers into new meals, such as turning vegetables into soups or using stale bread for croutons.

• **Practice portion control**: Serve smaller portions to reduce the amount of food that goes uneaten.

• **Store food properly**: Proper food storage can prolong the life of your produce and leftovers, reducing the likelihood of waste.

By incorporating these waste-free kitchen tips into your routine, you can significantly reduce the amount of food and packaging waste your household generates, leading to a more sustainable and responsible way of living.

To Keep In Mind: Reducing waste in your daily life doesn't require drastic changes—it's about making small, intentional choices that add up over time. From embracing the zero-waste movement and mindful consumption to upcycling and minimizing food waste, every effort counts. By adopting these practices, you'll contribute to a cleaner, healthier planet while inspiring others to join in the movement toward waste reduction and sustainability.

Chapter 3
Eco-Friendly Products and Packaging

As we become more conscious of the impact our choices have on the environment, it's essential to consider not only the products we buy but also their packaging. In this chapter, we will explore how to choose eco-friendly products, alternative packaging options, DIY solutions for cleaning and beauty, and tips to reduce single-use plastic consumption in your daily life.

Choosing Eco-Friendly Products: What to Look for in Household Items, Clothing, and Cosmetics

When shopping for household items, clothing, or cosmetics, it's important to be mindful of the environmental impact these products have. Eco-friendly products are made with sustainable materials, produced with minimal waste, and often designed to have a longer lifespan. Here's how to choose them:

1. Household Items:

• **Material Composition**: Look for items made from sustainable materials, such as bamboo, recycled metals, glass, or sustainably sourced wood. Avoid plastic, particularly products that are not recyclable or contain harmful chemicals like BPA.

• **Durability**: Choose durable and reusable products, such as stainless steel straws, reusable cleaning cloths, or wooden brushes, which are built to last and can replace disposable plastic alternatives.

• **Non-toxic**: Check for non-toxic finishes, paints, and materials that are free from harmful chemicals like phthalates and formaldehyde.

2. Clothing:

• **Sustainable Fabrics**: Look for clothing made from organic cotton, hemp, linen, or bamboo, which have a lower environmental impact compared to conventional cotton or synthetic fabrics. Avoid fast fashion and choose garments from ethical brands that focus on quality over quantity.

• **Certifications**: Look for certifications such as GOTS (Global Organic Textile Standard) or OEKO-TEX, which ensure that fabrics are produced sustainably and are free from harmful chemicals.

• **Second-Hand and Upcycled Fashion**: Embrace second-hand clothing or upcycled fashion to reduce the demand for new textiles and give old items a second life.

3. Cosmetics:

• **Natural Ingredients**: Choose cosmetics made with natural, organic, and cruelty-free ingredients. Avoid products that contain harmful chemicals such as parabens, phthalates, or artificial fragrances.

• **Eco-Friendly Packaging**: Opt for products packaged in recyclable or biodegradable materials like glass, metal, or paper instead of plastic.

• **Refillable Products**: Many cosmetics brands now offer refillable options for shampoos, lotions, and deodorants, allowing you to reuse the containers rather than constantly buying new ones.

By prioritizing these eco-friendly features, you'll help reduce the environmental impact of the products you buy while also supporting companies that are committed to sustainability.

Packaging Alternatives: Supporting Brands with Sustainable Packaging

Packaging waste, particularly plastic, is a significant contributor to environmental pollution. To reduce your impact, it's essential to choose brands that prioritize sustainable packaging options. Here's what to look for:

1. Minimalist Packaging:

• Choose brands that use the least amount of packaging possible. This includes packaging that is compact and doesn't rely on excessive layers or plastic wraps.

• Many brands are now adopting minimalist designs that reduce waste and make it easier to recycle.

2. Recyclable and Compostable Packaging:

• **Recyclable**: Look for packaging made from materials like glass, cardboard, or metal, which are more likely to be recyclable.

• **Compostable**: Some companies use plant-based or biodegradable materials for their packaging, such as compostable bags made from cornstarch or bamboo packaging. These materials break down naturally, reducing landfill waste.

3. Refill and Bulk Options:

• Some brands offer refillable packaging, allowing you to buy larger quantities of a product and refill the original container.

• Bulk shopping is another way to minimize packaging waste. Many stores now offer bulk bins for grains, nuts, cleaning supplies, and even personal care products.

4. Zero-Waste Packaging:

• Look for companies that are committed to zero-waste packaging. This means their products arrive without unnecessary plastic, and the packaging can either be recycled, composted, or reused. Some zero-waste brands even offer packaging-free products, such as shampoo bars, solid deodorants, and toothpaste tablets.

Supporting brands that prioritize sustainable packaging helps reduce plastic waste and encourages companies to invest in more eco-friendly alternatives.

DIY Solutions: How to Make Your Own Eco-Friendly Cleaning and Beauty Products

One of the easiest ways to reduce packaging waste and avoid harmful chemicals is by making your own cleaning and beauty products. DIY solutions are cost-effective, customizable, and better for the environment.

1. Eco-Friendly Cleaning Products: You can create a variety of cleaning solutions using simple, natural ingredients that are both effective and non-toxic.

• **All-Purpose Cleaner**: Mix equal parts water and white vinegar, with a few drops of essential oil (like lemon or tea tree oil) for a fresh scent. This solution can be used to clean countertops, glass, and floors.

• **Bathroom Cleaner**: Combine baking soda and vinegar to make a paste that can clean grout, sinks, and tubs. Add a few drops of essential oils for an extra fresh smell.

• **Dish Soap**: Melt a bar of natural soap (like Castile soap) and mix with water to create a gentle dish soap. Add essential oils or herbs for a pleasant fragrance.

2. Eco-Friendly Beauty Products: DIY beauty products are easy to make, free of synthetic chemicals, and reduce your reliance on plastic packaging.

• **Face Scrub**: Combine sugar or salt with coconut oil or honey to create a gentle exfoliating scrub.

• **Moisturizer**: Mix shea butter, coconut oil, and essential oils to make a rich, hydrating moisturizer.

• **Shampoo Bars**: You can create your own solid shampoo bars with natural ingredients like olive oil, coconut oil, and essential oils. These bars eliminate the need for plastic shampoo bottles.

• **Deodorant**: Mix coconut oil, baking soda, and cornstarch to make an effective, natural deodorant that you can store in a reusable jar.

By making your own products, you can avoid harmful chemicals and excessive packaging while tailoring each product to your specific needs.

Plastic-Free Living: Practical Tips to Reduce Single-Use Plastic Consumption

Plastic pollution is one of the most pressing environmental issues, particularly the rise of single-use plastics such as bottles, bags, and straws. Reducing plastic consumption is essential for protecting the planet's ecosystems and reducing waste. Here are practical tips for living a plastic-free life:

1. Choose Reusable Alternatives:

• **Water Bottles**: Invest in a high-quality reusable water bottle to eliminate the need for single-use plastic bottles.

• **Shopping Bags**: Carry your own reusable shopping bags made from cloth, jute, or other sustainable materials.

• **Straws**: Say no to plastic straws and opt for reusable alternatives made of stainless steel, glass, or bamboo.

• **Coffee Cups**: Bring your own reusable coffee cup or thermos when buying coffee to avoid disposable cups and lids.

2. Avoid Plastic Packaging:

• **Buy in Bulk**: Purchase food and household products in bulk, which often come with less packaging and allow you to use your own containers.

• **Choose Plastic-Free Brands**: Support companies that offer plastic-free products or packaging made from materials like glass, metal, or cardboard.

3. Make Conscious Choices:

• **Products with Minimal Packaging**: Look for products that are minimally packaged or use compostable materials. Avoid items that are heavily wrapped in plastic or include plastic-based packaging.

• **Second-Hand and Upcycled Goods**: Buying second-hand items and upcycled products can help reduce demand for new plastic goods.

4. Recycle Properly:

• **Sort Your Recycling**: Ensure that plastic items are disposed of properly by following local recycling guidelines. Avoid contamination by rinsing containers before recycling.

• **Avoid Non-Recyclable Plastics**: Some plastics are not recyclable, such as single-use plastics or plastic bags. Make sure you're aware of which plastics are accepted by your local recycling program.

To Keep In Mind: Adopting an eco-friendly lifestyle involves making thoughtful choices about the products you buy and the packaging they come in. By supporting brands with sustainable practices, opting for DIY solutions, and reducing single-use plastic consumption, you can significantly reduce your environmental footprint. With small, conscious changes, we can all contribute to a cleaner, healthier planet while enjoying eco-friendly products that align with our values.

Chapter 4
Sustainable Eating and Food Choices

Food choices play a significant role in environmental sustainability. From the resources used to grow, produce, and transport food to the waste generated from excess consumption, our diets can have a major impact on the planet. In this chapter, we will explore the benefits of plant-based diets, the importance of supporting local and seasonal foods, how to reduce food waste, and tips for sustainable grocery shopping.

Plant-Based Diets and Their Benefits: Why Shifting Toward Plant-Based Meals Can Reduce Your Carbon Footprint

One of the most effective ways to reduce your environmental impact is by shifting toward a plant-based diet. Animal agriculture is a leading contributor to environmental issues like deforestation, water pollution, and greenhouse gas emissions. By opting for plant-based meals, you can help mitigate these issues while also reaping personal health benefits.

Environmental Benefits of a Plant-Based Diet:

• **Lower Greenhouse Gas Emissions**: Producing plant-based foods generally results in fewer greenhouse gas emissions compared to raising livestock. Animal farming contributes significantly to methane emissions, a potent greenhouse gas.

• **Reduced Water Usage**: It takes far less water to grow plant-based foods than to raise animals. For example, producing one kilogram of beef requires approximately 15,000 liters of water, whereas producing the same amount of grains or vegetables may require just a few hundred liters.

• **Less Land Degradation**: Animal agriculture requires large amounts of land for grazing and growing feed crops. Shifting to plant-based diets reduces the demand for land and helps protect natural ecosystems.

• **Biodiversity Preservation**: Large-scale livestock farming is a major driver of deforestation and habitat loss, leading to a decline in biodiversity. A plant-based diet can help reduce the pressure on forests and wildlife.

Health Benefits of Plant-Based Eating:

• **Improved Health**: Plant-based diets are often rich in vitamins, minerals, and fiber while being lower in saturated fats, which can help reduce the risk of chronic diseases like heart disease, diabetes, and obesity.

• **Weight Management**: Many plant-based foods are nutrient-dense and lower in calories, making them an excellent choice for maintaining a healthy weight.

How to Start:

• **Meatless Days**: Try introducing one or more meatless days a week (e.g., Meatless Monday) to ease into a plant-based diet.

- **Explore Plant-Based Proteins**: Incorporate plant-based proteins like beans, lentils, tofu, tempeh, quinoa, and seitan into your meals.

- **Eat More Whole Foods**: Focus on whole, minimally processed plant foods such as vegetables, fruits, whole grains, nuts, and seeds.

By shifting towards a plant-based diet, you can dramatically reduce your carbon footprint and contribute to a healthier planet.

Supporting Local and Seasonal Foods: How Buying Local Produce Supports Sustainability

Buying local and seasonal foods offers numerous environmental and community benefits. Local produce typically has a smaller carbon footprint because it doesn't have to be transported long distances, and seasonal foods are grown in harmony with nature's cycles, reducing the need for artificial inputs like pesticides and fertilizers.

Benefits of Supporting Local and Seasonal Foods:

- **Reduced Carbon Footprint**: Locally grown food doesn't need to be shipped across the country or internationally, which significantly reduces the environmental impact from transportation.

- **Support for Local Farmers**: Buying local produce supports small-scale farmers and keeps money circulating within local economies.

- **Fresher, More Nutritious Produce**: Local and seasonal foods are often fresher than those transported from far away. Fresher food typically retains more nutrients and tastes better.

• **Less Packaging**: Locally grown produce often comes with minimal packaging, which reduces waste compared to supermarket produce that may be wrapped in plastic.

How to Incorporate More Local and Seasonal Foods:

• **Visit Farmers' Markets**: Farmers' markets are a great place to find fresh, seasonal produce and reduce your food's carbon footprint.

• **Join a CSA (Community Supported Agriculture)**: CSAs allow you to buy a share of a local farm's produce. This helps support local farmers and ensures you're eating food grown near you.

• **Grow Your Own**: If you have the space, try growing your own fruits and vegetables. Homegrown food eliminates transportation emissions and offers the satisfaction of knowing where your food comes from.

By making local and seasonal foods a priority, you contribute to sustainable agriculture practices and help preserve the environment.

Reducing Food Waste: Tips on Meal Planning and Smart Storage to Avoid Food Waste

Food waste is a major environmental issue, with millions of tons of food thrown away each year. Not only does this waste contribute to landfill overflow, but it also represents wasted resources, including water, energy, and labor. Fortunately, there are many ways to reduce food waste through careful planning, smart storage, and creative use of leftovers.

How to Reduce Food Waste:

• **Meal Planning**: Plan your meals for the week to avoid buying excessive amounts of food. Write down a shopping list and stick to it to prevent impulse purchases that could go unused.

• **Portion Control**: Serve smaller portions to avoid cooking more than you can eat. Leftovers can be stored and used in future meals, minimizing waste.

• **Use Leftovers Creatively**: Repurpose leftovers into new meals—use vegetables from last night's dinner in soups, salads, or stir-fries, or transform leftover grains into a grain bowl or fried rice.

• **Freeze Leftovers**: Freeze food that won't be used in time. This is a great way to preserve produce, grains, or cooked meals and reduce the chances of food spoiling.

• **Compost Food Scraps**: Compost fruit and vegetable scraps, coffee grounds, and eggshells. This creates nutrient-rich soil for your garden, reducing landfill waste and giving back to the earth.

Smart Storage Tips:

• **Properly Store Produce**: Some fruits and vegetables last longer when stored in the fridge, while others should be kept at room temperature. Research how to store different foods to maximize their shelf life.

• **Use Glass Containers**: Store leftovers and prepared meals in glass containers instead of plastic. Glass keeps food fresh and avoids harmful chemicals from leaching into your food.

• **Keep Track of Expiration Dates**: Organize your pantry and fridge to ensure older items are used first. Check expiration dates regularly and rotate items to avoid wasting food.

By reducing food waste, you conserve valuable resources and

decrease the environmental impact associated with food production and disposal.

Sustainable Grocery Shopping: How to Shop Responsibly and Avoid Plastic-Wrapped Products

When you're grocery shopping, the choices you make can have a lasting impact on the environment. From avoiding plastic-wrapped products to supporting sustainable brands, there are several ways to shop responsibly and reduce waste.

Tips for Sustainable Grocery Shopping:

• **Bring Your Own Bags**: Always carry reusable shopping bags to avoid using plastic bags. You can also use reusable mesh produce bags for fruits and vegetables.

• **Shop in Bulk**: Buying bulk items reduces packaging waste. Many stores offer bulk bins for grains, nuts, seeds, pasta, and even cleaning products. Bring your own containers or bags to fill.

• **Avoid Pre-Packaged Produce**: Skip the pre-packaged fruits and vegetables wrapped in plastic. Instead, buy loose produce and place them in reusable bags.

• **Support Ethical Brands**: Choose products from brands that focus on sustainability, ethical sourcing, and eco-friendly packaging. Look for certifications like Fair Trade, Organic, and B Corp.

• **Buy Organic When Possible**: Organic farming practices tend to be more environmentally friendly, avoiding synthetic pesticides and fertilizers and promoting soil health.

How to Avoid Plastic-Wrapped Products:

• **Choose Glass or Paper Packaging**: Opt for products

packaged in glass, metal, or paper, which are more easily recyclable than plastic.

• **Opt for Frozen Over Fresh**: Fresh produce may come in plastic packaging, but frozen produce often has less packaging or uses more eco-friendly alternatives.

By shopping consciously and avoiding plastic-wrapped products, you help reduce plastic waste and support businesses that are committed to sustainable practices.

To Keep In Mind: Sustainable eating and food choices are essential for reducing your environmental impact and promoting long-term planetary health. By shifting toward plant-based meals, supporting local and seasonal foods, reducing food waste, and shopping responsibly, you can make a significant difference in your carbon footprint. Every conscious choice you make in the kitchen contributes to a more sustainable food system and a healthier planet for generations to come.

Chapter 5
Eco-Friendly Transportation

Transportation is a significant contributor to greenhouse gas emissions, with cars, trucks, and airplanes being major sources of pollution. However, there are numerous ways to reduce your carbon footprint when it comes to getting around. This chapter will explore sustainable travel options, the benefits of electric and hybrid vehicles, carpooling and ride-sharing, and how carbon offsetting can help balance out emissions from your travel.

Choosing Sustainable Travel Options: Walking, Cycling, and Public Transport

One of the easiest and most effective ways to reduce your carbon footprint is by choosing alternative modes of transportation that have minimal environmental impact. Walking, cycling, and public transport are all sustainable options that not only help the environment but also promote personal health and well-being.

1. Walking:

• **No Emissions**: Walking is the most eco-friendly way to travel since it involves no emissions at all.

- **Health Benefits**: Walking improves cardiovascular health, reduces stress, and is a simple way to get more exercise into your daily routine.

- **Practical for Short Distances**: Walking is ideal for short trips, such as running errands, commuting to work or school, or visiting nearby friends and family.

2. Cycling:

- **Low Carbon Footprint**: Cycling is another zero-emissions transportation option that is more efficient than walking, particularly for slightly longer distances.

- **Health and Fitness**: Cycling provides an excellent cardiovascular workout and can be an enjoyable way to stay fit and reduce stress.

- **Cost-Effective**: Once you've invested in a bicycle, it costs very little to maintain, making it a highly cost-effective mode of transport.

- **Bicycle-Friendly Cities**: Many cities around the world are investing in cycling infrastructure, making it easier and safer to use bicycles for daily commuting.

3. Public Transport:

- **Reduced Traffic and Emissions**: Taking public transportation, such as buses, trams, or trains, reduces the number of individual vehicles on the road, lowering congestion and emissions.

- **Cost-Effective**: Public transport is often cheaper than owning a car, especially when considering the cost of fuel, insurance, and maintenance.

• **Wide Accessibility**: In urban areas, public transport is often an efficient and reliable option for daily commuting. It also helps reduce the need for parking, which is both costly and space-consuming in cities.

Choosing to walk, cycle, or use public transport whenever possible can significantly reduce your environmental impact and improve your quality of life.

Electric and Hybrid Vehicles: The Environmental Benefits of Greener Car Choices

While walking, cycling, and public transport are great choices, there are still times when driving is necessary. If you must drive, opting for electric or hybrid vehicles is an effective way to reduce your carbon footprint while still getting around in a car.

1. Electric Vehicles (EVs):

• **Zero Emissions**: EVs run entirely on electricity, producing no tailpipe emissions, unlike traditional gasoline or diesel-powered vehicles. This helps reduce air pollution, particularly in urban areas.

• **Energy Efficiency**: Electric cars are much more energy-efficient than internal combustion engine (ICE) vehicles, using less energy to travel the same distance.

• **Cost Savings**: While the initial purchase price of an EV can be higher than a traditional car, the long-term costs are lower due to savings on fuel (electricity is generally cheaper than gasoline) and reduced maintenance (EVs have fewer moving parts than gas-powered cars).

• **Incentives and Support**: Many governments offer financial incentives, rebates, and tax credits for purchasing EVs, making them more affordable. Additionally, there are growing networks of charging stations, making EVs more convenient for long-distance travel.

2. Hybrid Vehicles:

• **Dual Power Sources**: Hybrid cars combine an internal combustion engine with an electric motor. This allows the vehicle to run on electricity at low speeds and switch to gasoline for longer trips, which reduces overall fuel consumption and emissions.

• **Fuel Efficiency**: Hybrids are more fuel-efficient than traditional gasoline cars, helping to reduce both greenhouse gas emissions and your reliance on fossil fuels.

• **Lower Operating Costs**: Like EVs, hybrid vehicles generally have lower maintenance costs than conventional cars, and they save you money on fuel in the long term.

Switching to electric or hybrid vehicles is a great way to make your travel more sustainable while still enjoying the convenience of car ownership.

Carpooling and Ride-Sharing: How to Reduce Your Carbon Footprint When Traveling

Carpooling and ride-sharing are excellent ways to reduce the number of vehicles on the road, cutting down on both traffic congestion and emissions. By sharing rides with others, you can lower your personal carbon footprint while also saving money on fuel and parking.

1. Carpooling:

• **Shared Rides**: Carpooling involves sharing a ride with others who are traveling in the same direction. This reduces the number of cars on the road and can significantly lower your emissions per trip.

• **Cost Savings**: Carpooling allows you to share the costs of fuel and parking with other passengers, making it an affordable way to travel.

• **Convenience**: Many areas offer carpool lanes, which allow you to bypass traffic and arrive at your destination faster.

2. Ride-Sharing:

• **Ride-Share Services**: Platforms like Uber, Lyft, and others allow you to share a ride with someone else who is going in the same direction. This reduces the number of vehicles on the road and offers a convenient, often cheaper alternative to traditional taxi services.

• **Electric and Hybrid Options**: Some ride-sharing services offer electric or hybrid vehicle options, further reducing the environmental impact of your travel.

• **Pooling Rides**: Most ride-sharing services also allow you to opt for "pooling" options, where you share the ride with other passengers, maximizing the number of people per car and reducing emissions.

Carpooling and ride-sharing can make a big difference in reducing your personal carbon footprint, especially for people who need to travel long distances for work, school, or other activities.

Offsetting Carbon Emissions: What Is Carbon Offsetting, and How Can It Work for You?

Even with all the sustainable transportation choices available, some travel—particularly air travel—produces significant carbon emissions. Carbon offsetting is a way to neutralize those emissions by investing in projects that reduce or capture greenhouse gases elsewhere.

1. What Is Carbon Offsetting? Carbon offsetting involves purchasing credits that fund projects designed to reduce, capture, or prevent greenhouse gas emissions. These projects can include reforestation (planting trees), renewable energy installations (such as wind and solar), and methane capture from landfills.

2. How Carbon Offsetting Works:

• **Calculation**: Many carbon offset programs allow you to calculate the carbon emissions from a specific activity (e.g., a flight or a road trip) and then purchase offsets equivalent to that amount of carbon.

• **Support for Environmental Projects**: The money from carbon offset purchases goes toward projects that work to reduce or eliminate carbon emissions, such as forest conservation, clean energy development, or methane capture.

3. When to Use Carbon Offsetting:

• **Air Travel**: Flights are one of the most carbon-intensive forms of travel. Carbon offsetting can help balance out the emissions generated by your flight, contributing to projects that reduce greenhouse gases.

• **Long-Distance Car Travel**: If you have to drive a long distance or rent a car, you can offset your vehicle's emissions by purchasing credits from offset programs.

4. Choosing an Offset Program:

• **Verified Projects**: Ensure the offset program supports verified, high-quality projects. Look for certifications such as the Gold Standard or the Verified Carbon Standard (VCS) to ensure the projects are legitimate and effective.

- **Transparency**: Choose programs that provide clear information about how your money is being used and the specific projects being funded.

While carbon offsetting doesn't negate the importance of reducing emissions at the source, it can be a useful tool for neutralizing emissions from travel and supporting global efforts to combat climate change.

To Keep In Mind: Eco-friendly transportation is a key aspect of sustainable living. By choosing sustainable travel options like walking, cycling, and public transport, investing in electric or hybrid vehicles, and embracing carpooling or ride-sharing, you can reduce your environmental impact and contribute to a greener planet. Additionally, carbon offsetting offers a way to neutralize unavoidable emissions from activities like air travel. Each choice you make regarding transportation can help you live more sustainably and reduce your carbon footprint.

Chapter 6
Energy Conservation at Home

Energy consumption is one of the largest contributors to environmental degradation, with homes accounting for a significant portion of global energy use. By making simple yet impactful changes in how we use energy at home, we can reduce our carbon footprint and save money. This chapter explores how to choose energy-efficient appliances, reduce home energy use, explore renewable energy options, and leverage smart home technologies to save energy.

Energy-Efficient Appliances: How to Choose and Use Them Effectively

Energy-efficient appliances are designed to use less energy while performing the same tasks as traditional models. By choosing energy-efficient appliances, you can reduce your energy consumption, lower utility bills, and contribute to environmental sustainability.

1. What to Look for in Energy-Efficient Appliances:

• **Energy Star Certification**: Look for the Energy Star label, which indicates that an appliance meets energy efficiency standards set by the U.S. Environmental Protection Agency (EPA). These appliances consume less energy and have a lower environmental impact.

• **High Efficiency Ratings**: Check for high efficiency ratings in specific appliances. For example, washing machines with high spin speeds use less water and energy, while refrigerators with better insulation consume less electricity.

• **Size Appropriateness**: Choose appliances that are appropriately sized for your needs. A larger appliance than necessary, such as an oversized refrigerator or air conditioner, uses more energy than required.

2. Tips for Using Appliances Efficiently:

• **Use the Right Settings**: Many appliances, like dishwashers, washing machines, and ovens, have energy-saving settings that you can use to reduce energy consumption.

• **Regular Maintenance**: Maintain your appliances properly to ensure they operate efficiently. Clean filters, coils, and vents to optimize their energy use and prolong their lifespan.

• **Turn Off When Not in Use**: Unplug appliances when not in use or use a power strip to easily disconnect several devices at once, reducing "phantom" or "standby" energy use.

By selecting energy-efficient appliances and using them wisely, you can significantly reduce your home's energy consumption and contribute to a more sustainable lifestyle.

Reducing Home Energy Use: Simple Steps Like Using LED Bulbs and Insulating Your Home

There are several simple, cost-effective ways to reduce your energy use at home. These steps can have an immediate impact on your electricity consumption and, in turn, your utility bills.

1. Switch to LED Bulbs:

• **Energy Efficiency**: LED bulbs use at least 75% less energy than incandescent bulbs, and they last much longer. This means less energy is consumed to produce light, and fewer bulbs are disposed of over time.

• **Improved Lighting**: LED bulbs provide bright, clear light without generating excess heat, which can make your home more comfortable and reduce cooling needs in warmer months.

2. Insulate Your Home:

• **Heat Retention**: Proper insulation helps keep your home warm in the winter and cool in the summer by reducing heat transfer. This means your heating and cooling systems work less, reducing energy consumption.

• **Sealing Gaps**: Check for gaps around windows, doors, and vents. Use caulking and weatherstripping to seal any leaks, preventing warm or cool air from escaping.

• **Attic and Wall Insulation**: Insulating your attic, walls, and floors can further reduce energy loss, improving comfort and reducing heating and cooling costs year-round.

3. Optimize Heating and Cooling:

• **Programmable Thermostats**: Set your thermostat to automatically adjust the temperature based on when you are home or away. Lowering the temperature by a few degrees in winter or raising it in summer can significantly save energy.

• **Ceiling Fans**: In the summer, use ceiling fans to circulate air, which can make you feel cooler and reduce the need for air conditioning.

• **Regular Maintenance**: Ensure that your HVAC system is well-maintained, including changing filters and servicing the system to ensure it operates efficiently.

4. Reduce Water Heating Costs:

• **Lower Water Heater Temperature**: Lower the temperature of your water heater to 120°F (49°C). This helps reduce energy use and can prevent scalding.

• **Insulate Water Heater and Pipes**: Insulate your water heater and pipes to retain heat, making it more energy-efficient.

By taking these steps to reduce your home's energy use, you can make a meaningful impact on both the environment and your wallet.

Renewable Energy Options: Solar, Wind, and Other Sustainable Energy Sources

Renewable energy sources are clean, sustainable, and can provide your home with energy without contributing to climate change. Although the upfront cost of installation can be high, renewable energy systems often pay off in the long run by reducing utility bills and increasing home value.

1. Solar Power:

• **Photovoltaic (PV) Panels**: Solar panels convert sunlight into electricity, providing a clean, renewable energy source. By installing solar panels on your roof, you can generate your own electricity, reducing your reliance on fossil fuels.

• **Net Metering**: Some utility companies offer net metering programs that allow you to sell excess energy back to the grid, which can offset your installation costs and make your solar investment more economical.

• **Solar Water Heating**: Solar thermal systems can be used to heat water for your home. These systems use solar panels to absorb heat and transfer it to water, which can reduce the need for electric or gas water heaters.

2. Wind Power:

• **Residential Wind Turbines**: If you live in a location with consistent wind, installing a small residential wind turbine can generate electricity. These turbines can be used in combination with solar power systems or independently.

• **Off-Grid or Grid-Tied**: Wind power systems can be connected to the grid to provide energy to your home or used off-grid to power a remote cabin or property.

3. Geothermal Energy:

• **Geothermal Heat Pumps**: Geothermal energy harnesses the heat from beneath the Earth's surface to provide heating and cooling for your home. A geothermal heat pump system can significantly reduce energy costs by providing efficient, sustainable climate control.

4. Biomass Energy:

• **Wood Stoves and Biomass Heating Systems**: Biomass systems burn organic materials (such as wood pellets) to generate heat or electricity. This can be a sustainable heating option if the wood is sourced responsibly from renewable forests.

By investing in renewable energy options, you can reduce your reliance on non-renewable resources and contribute to a cleaner, greener future.

Smart Home Technologies: How Smart Thermostats and Energy Monitoring Can Help Save Energy

Smart home technologies have revolutionized the way we manage energy use at home. These devices offer convenience and control, helping you reduce energy consumption without sacrificing comfort.

1. Smart Thermostats:

• **Automated Temperature Control**: Smart thermostats like Nest and Ecobee allow you to set schedules for your heating and cooling systems, ensuring they only operate when necessary. You can also control the temperature remotely via smartphone apps, saving energy when you're away.

• **Learning Your Patterns**: Some smart thermostats learn your daily patterns and adjust automatically to optimize energy use. For example, they might lower the temperature when you leave for work and raise it just before you return.

• **Energy Reports**: Many smart thermostats provide energy reports, helping you monitor your usage and find areas where you can save.

2. Energy Monitoring Systems:

• **Real-Time Energy Tracking**: Devices like Sense and EnergyHub allow you to monitor your home's energy consumption in real-time. These systems can identify which appliances or devices are using the most energy, helping you make adjustments to reduce waste.

• **Integration with Other Smart Devices**: Energy monitoring systems can integrate with smart plugs and appliances, allowing you to automate energy-saving actions (e.g., turning off appliances when not in use).

3. Smart Lighting:

• **Motion-Sensing and Dimming**: Smart lighting systems automatically turn off when no motion is detected, and many also allow you to adjust the brightness based on the time of day or your preferences. Dimming lights when full brightness isn't needed can reduce energy use.

• **App-Controlled**: Some smart bulbs can be controlled via smartphone apps or voice assistants like Alexa or Google Assistant, giving you full control over your lighting even when you're away from home.

4. Smart Appliances:

• **Energy-Efficient Choices**: Many smart appliances, such as refrigerators, washers, and dryers, come with energy-saving modes and allow you to monitor their energy usage. They can also be scheduled to run during off-peak hours, reducing your electricity costs.

Smart home technologies help you optimize energy consumption, reduce waste, and ultimately save money by giving you better control over how and when your appliances use energy.

To Keep In Mind: Energy conservation at home is an essential part of living sustainably. By choosing energy-efficient appliances, reducing energy use through simple measures like LED bulbs and insulation, exploring renewable energy options like solar and wind power, and leveraging smart home technologies, you can significantly reduce your home's energy consumption. Not only will this lower your carbon footprint, but it will also save you money in the long term. Taking action to conserve energy today will help create a more sustainable future for both your family and the planet.

Chapter 7
Water Conservation Tips

Water is a vital resource for life, yet it is becoming increasingly scarce in many parts of the world. The demand for clean water is rising, while the supply is limited by droughts, pollution, and climate change. Conserving water is essential to ensure a sustainable future for both the environment and human populations. In this chapter, we will explore the water crisis, provide tips for reducing water waste, and offer solutions like rainwater harvesting to help you conserve water in your daily life.

The Water Crisis: Why Conserving Water is Crucial for the Environment

Water scarcity is a growing global issue, and by 2025, it's estimated that nearly two-thirds of the world's population could face water shortages. Here are some key reasons why water conservation is critical:

1. Increasing Demand:

• Global population growth, industrialization, and agricultural expansion are putting increasing pressure on available freshwater resources. Many regions already rely on unsustainable levels of water extraction, further exacerbating the crisis.

2. Climate Change:

• Climate change is leading to more severe weather patterns, such as prolonged droughts and unpredictable rainfall. In some areas, water resources are being depleted faster than they can be replenished by natural processes.

3. Ecosystem Impact:

• Freshwater ecosystems, such as rivers, lakes, and wetlands, are critical habitats for many species. Overuse of water can harm these ecosystems, leading to a loss of biodiversity and the degradation of essential environmental functions.

4. Energy Use and Water:

• The production and transportation of water require a significant amount of energy. Conserving water also reduces the energy used for water treatment and delivery, which can help reduce overall carbon emissions.

By conserving water, we can help protect natural ecosystems, reduce the energy used for water treatment, and ensure that future generations have access to the water they need to thrive.

Low-Water Solutions: Installing Water-Saving Devices Like Low-Flow Showerheads and Faucets

One of the easiest ways to conserve water in your home is by installing water-saving devices that reduce water consumption without sacrificing comfort or convenience. These devices are designed to use less water while still delivering the performance you need.

1. Low-Flow Showerheads:

• **Water-Saving Technology**: Low-flow showerheads use air to mix with the water, creating the sensation of higher water pressure without using excess water. Modern low-flow showerheads can use as little as 1.5 to 2 gallons of water per minute, compared to the 5 gallons per minute that traditional showerheads often use.

• **Energy Savings**: Since water heating accounts for a significant portion of home energy use, reducing the amount of hot water you use in the shower can lower both your water and energy bills.

2. Low-Flow Faucets:

• **Efficient Design**: Low-flow faucets and aerators regulate the flow of water, reducing the amount used while maintaining a good water pressure. They can reduce water flow to 1.5 gallons per minute (gpm), compared to 2.2 gpm or more for standard faucets.

• **Easy Installation**: Installing low-flow faucets is an easy and affordable DIY project that can yield significant savings on both water and energy bills over time.

3. Water-Saving Toilets:

• **Dual-Flush Systems**: Toilets with dual-flush systems allow you to choose between a low-volume flush for liquid waste and a higher-volume flush for solid waste. This helps conserve water without sacrificing performance.

• **High-Efficiency Toilets (HETs)**: These toilets use as little as 1.28 gallons per flush, compared to traditional toilets that use 3.5 to 7 gallons per flush.

By upgrading your fixtures to low-water options, you can conserve a significant amount of water each year, making a positive impact on both your home's water use and your utility bills.

Mindful Water Use: Simple Practices for Reducing Water Waste

In addition to installing water-saving devices, adopting mindful water use practices in your daily life can help reduce unnecessary water consumption.

1. Fix Leaks Promptly:

• **Hidden Water Waste**: Leaky faucets, pipes, and toilets can waste large amounts of water over time. A leaking faucet can waste as much as 3,000 gallons of water per year, while a running toilet can waste up to 200 gallons a day.

• **Simple Repairs**: Most leaks can be fixed with basic tools and a little know-how. Regularly check for leaks in your plumbing, and promptly repair any issues to prevent water waste.

2. Take Shorter Showers:

• **Reduce Time in the Shower**: Reducing the amount of time you spend in the shower can significantly cut down on water use. Consider setting a timer or challenging yourself to limit shower time to 5 minutes.

• **Turn Off While Lathering**: Turn off the water while you lather soap or shampoo, and only turn it back on when you need to rinse. This simple practice can save gallons of water per shower.

3. Full Loads Only:

• **Dishwasher and Laundry**: Only run the dishwasher or washing machine when they are full to maximize water efficiency. Running these appliances with partial loads wastes water and energy.

• **Optimize Settings**: Use eco-friendly settings on your washing machine and dishwasher to reduce water use. Many modern appliances have specific settings that use less water while still cleaning effectively.

4. Use a Bucket for Washing Cars:

• **Avoid the Hose**: Instead of using a running hose to wash your car, use a bucket and sponge. A hose can use up to 8 gallons of water per minute, while a bucket can help you limit water use to only what is needed.

5. Water Plants Wisely:

• **Early Morning or Late Evening**: Water your plants during cooler parts of the day, such as early morning or late evening, to prevent water evaporation. This ensures your plants get the moisture they need while minimizing waste.

• **Water Efficiently**: Use a watering can or drip irrigation system to deliver water directly to the roots, rather than spraying it from a hose, which can result in excessive evaporation.

Being mindful of everyday water use and making small changes can lead to significant reductions in your overall water consumption.

Rainwater Harvesting: How to Collect and Use Rainwater for Landscaping

Rainwater harvesting is the process of collecting and storing rainwater for later use, primarily for landscaping and irrigation purposes. This practice not only reduces your water bill but also helps conserve potable water for essential uses.

1. Setting Up a Rainwater Harvesting System:

• **Gutter System**: Start by installing gutters and downspouts that direct rainwater into a storage container, such as a rain barrel or large water tank. Ensure the system is properly filtered to remove debris before water enters the storage container.

• **Storage Capacity**: Choose a rainwater storage system that fits your needs. Smaller rain barrels can hold 50-100 gallons, while larger systems can store thousands of gallons.

• **Pump and Irrigation**: For larger gardens or lawns, you can install a pump to move water from the storage tank to your plants through a drip irrigation system. This is a highly efficient way to water your garden, using rainwater instead of treated tap water.

2. Benefits of Rainwater Harvesting:

• **Environmental Benefits**: Rainwater harvesting reduces the demand on municipal water systems and helps reduce stormwater runoff, which can cause erosion and pollution.

• **Cost Savings**: By using rainwater for landscaping, you can significantly reduce the amount of water you use from the tap, resulting in lower water bills.

• **Chemical-Free Water**: Rainwater is naturally soft and free of the chemicals, like chlorine and fluoride, that are often found in tap water. This makes it ideal for watering plants, as it's gentler on the soil and more beneficial for plant health.

3. Legal Considerations:

• **Check Local Regulations**: In some regions, rainwater harvesting may be regulated or even restricted, so it's important to check local laws before setting up a system.

Rainwater harvesting is a sustainable practice that can help reduce water use for landscaping, particularly in dry climates where water conservation is especially important.

To Keep In Mind: Water conservation is an essential component of sustainable living. By installing low-water devices, being mindful of daily water use, fixing leaks, and collecting rainwater, you can significantly reduce your water consumption. These changes not only help conserve this precious resource but also save you money on your utility bills. Every small action you take toward water conservation helps protect the environment, ensures clean water for future generations, and supports global efforts to address water scarcity.

Chapter 8
Sustainable Fashion

The fashion industry is one of the largest contributors to environmental pollution, with fast fashion driving mass production, overconsumption, and significant waste. However, as consumers become more aware of the environmental impact of their choices, sustainable fashion has emerged as a solution. By choosing quality over quantity, supporting eco-friendly materials, and embracing practices like second-hand shopping and clothing repair, we can all contribute to a more sustainable future. This chapter will explore the concept of slow fashion, eco-friendly fabrics, how to refresh your wardrobe without buying new, and how to care for and repair your clothes to extend their lifespan.

Slow Fashion: Why Choosing Quality Over Fast Fashion Makes a Difference

Fast fashion is characterized by mass-producing cheap, trendy clothing that is designed to be worn a few times before being discarded. This model promotes overconsumption, textile waste, and labor exploitation, all of which contribute to environmental degradation.

1. Environmental Impact of Fast Fashion:

• **Resource Intensity**: The fast fashion industry consumes large amounts of water, energy, and raw materials. For example, it can take around 2,700 liters of water to make one cotton t-shirt, which is equivalent to the amount of water a person drinks over the course of 2.5 years.

• **Waste and Pollution**: Fast fashion leads to a significant amount of textile waste. The average American discards about 70 pounds of clothing each year, with much of it ending up in landfills. Moreover, the production processes often involve toxic chemicals that pollute the air, water, and soil.

• **Poor Quality**: Fast fashion garments are often made from low-quality materials and designed to last for only one or two seasons. As a result, they are discarded more quickly, contributing to an unsustainable cycle of overproduction and overconsumption.

2. Benefits of Slow Fashion:

• **Quality Over Quantity**: Slow fashion encourages consumers to invest in fewer, high-quality pieces that will last longer. This reduces the need for constant replacement and lowers the overall environmental footprint.

• **Timeless Pieces**: Slow fashion emphasizes classic styles that never go out of fashion, reducing the pressure to keep up with ever-changing trends.

• **Ethical Production**: Many slow fashion brands prioritize fair labor practices, sustainable sourcing, and transparency in their supply chains.

By embracing slow fashion, we can make more thoughtful purchasing decisions that support ethical labor practices, reduce waste, and lower our environmental impact.

Eco-Friendly Fabrics: What Fabrics to Look For and Avoid

The materials used in clothing have a significant environmental impact. Choosing fabrics that are sustainably produced, biodegradable, or recycled can reduce the harm caused by clothing production.

1. Sustainable Fabrics to Look For:

• **Organic Cotton**: Unlike conventional cotton, organic cotton is grown without synthetic pesticides or fertilizers, which reduces soil and water contamination. Organic cotton farming also uses fewer resources and supports biodiversity.

• **Hemp**: Hemp is a highly sustainable fabric because it requires little water, no pesticides, and grows quickly. It is also durable and biodegradable, making it an excellent alternative to cotton.

• **Linen**: Made from the flax plant, linen is biodegradable, requires fewer pesticides and water than cotton, and has a low environmental impact. It is also a durable and breathable fabric, ideal for warm climates.

• **Tencel (Lyocell)**: Tencel is made from sustainably harvested wood pulp, primarily from eucalyptus, beech, or spruce trees. The production process uses a closed-loop system, where solvents are recycled, reducing waste and pollution.

• **Recycled Fabrics**: Fabrics made from recycled materials, such as polyester made from post-consumer plastic bottles or recycled wool, help reduce the need for virgin resources and reduce waste.

2. Fabrics to Avoid:

• **Conventional Cotton**: While cotton is a natural fiber, conventional cotton farming uses large amounts of pesticides and fertilizers, which are harmful to the environment and human health. It also requires a significant amount of water, contributing to water scarcity in certain regions.

• **Polyester and Other Synthetics**: Polyester, nylon, and acrylic are petroleum-based fabrics that are not biodegradable. They shed microplastics into the environment during washing, polluting water systems and harming marine life.

• **Leather**: Traditional leather production is resource-intensive and involves toxic chemicals like chromium, which can pollute water systems and harm ecosystems. Alternatives like plant-based or lab-grown leather are more sustainable options.

By choosing fabrics that are sustainably sourced, biodegradable, or recycled, we can reduce the environmental impact of our clothing choices.

Clothing Swaps and Second-Hand Shopping: How to Refresh Your Wardrobe Without Buying New

One of the best ways to reduce your environmental footprint in fashion is by buying less new clothing. Clothing swaps and second-hand shopping allow you to refresh your wardrobe while extending the life of pre-loved garments.

1. Clothing Swaps:

• **How It Works**: Clothing swaps are community events where people exchange gently used clothing items. They are a great way to refresh your wardrobe without contributing to the waste of fast fashion. You can find local clothing swap groups or organize your own with friends and family.

• **Benefits**: Clothing swaps prevent textiles from going to landfills, promote sustainable consumption, and often allow you to find unique pieces that aren't available in stores. It's also a fun way to connect with others while promoting sustainability.

2. Second-Hand Shopping:

• **Thrift Stores and Consignment Shops**: Thrift stores, second-hand shops, and consignment stores are treasure troves for pre-owned clothing. By shopping second-hand, you are reusing and repurposing clothing, which prevents it from being discarded prematurely.

• **Online Platforms**: Platforms like Depop, Poshmark, and ThredUp offer second-hand clothes in excellent condition, often from high-quality brands at a fraction of the cost. Shopping online second-hand is a convenient way to shop sustainably and find unique, vintage pieces.

• **Vintage and Upcycled Clothing**: Vintage shops and upcycled clothing brands offer curated selections of clothes with historical value or those that have been creatively repurposed. These garments often have a longer lifespan and more character than mass-produced fashion.

By choosing second-hand or swapping clothing, we can help reduce the demand for new garments and the resources required to make them.

Care and Repair: Extending the Life of Your Clothes Through Proper Care and Mending

One of the most sustainable things you can do for your wardrobe is to take care of the clothes you already own. By extending the life of your garments, you reduce waste and lessen the need for new clothing purchases.

1. Proper Care:

• **Washing Less Frequently**: Washing clothes uses water and energy, and frequent washing can wear out fabrics faster. Consider wearing clothes more than once before washing them, especially if they're not visibly dirty.

• **Cold Water and Air Drying**: Washing clothes in cold water reduces energy consumption. Air drying your clothes instead of using a dryer also conserves energy and helps extend the lifespan of fabrics.

• **Gentle Detergents**: Choose eco-friendly laundry detergents that are free of harsh chemicals, which can be harmful to both the environment and your clothes. Look for biodegradable options that are gentle on fabrics and the planet.

2. Repairing Clothes:

• **Mending Small Tears and Holes**: Simple repairs like sewing up small tears, replacing buttons, or patching up holes can extend the life of your garments by years. These skills are valuable and can help you reduce textile waste.

• **Dyeing and Upcycling**: If your clothes are looking worn or faded, consider dyeing them or upcycling them into something new, such as turning an old shirt into a tote bag. There are plenty of DIY guides online to help you get creative with your clothing.

3. Professional Repair Services:

• **Tailoring and Alterations**: Professional tailoring can help make your clothes last longer by altering them to fit better, fixing damaged zippers, or reinforcing areas that experience wear and tear. This can help you hold onto your favorite pieces for years to come.

Taking care of your clothes and repairing them when needed is one of the most effective ways to reduce the environmental impact of your wardrobe.

To Keep In Mind: Sustainable fashion is not just about buying eco-friendly clothing; it's about making thoughtful choices that prioritize quality, longevity, and ethical production. By embracing slow fashion, choosing sustainable fabrics, shopping second-hand, and extending the life of your clothes through proper care and repair, you can significantly reduce your impact on the planet. Small changes in how you approach fashion can lead to a more sustainable, ethical, and eco-friendly wardrobe, helping you contribute to a greener world one outfit at a time.

Chapter 9
Sustainable Gardening and Landscaping

Gardening is one of the most rewarding ways to embrace sustainability. Whether you have a small balcony garden or a large backyard, sustainable gardening practices can help you reduce your environmental footprint, support local ecosystems, and even provide fresh food. In this chapter, we will explore how growing your own food, supporting biodiversity through native plants and organic gardening, reducing water waste through efficient landscaping, and composting can all contribute to a greener, more sustainable lifestyle.

Benefits of Growing Your Own Food: How a Home Garden Can Contribute to a Sustainable Lifestyle

Growing your own food offers numerous environmental and personal benefits. It reduces the carbon footprint associated with food production and transportation, provides you with fresh and healthy produce, and strengthens your connection to nature.

1. Environmental Benefits:

• **Reducing Food Miles**: Commercially grown produce often travels long distances to reach your table, contributing to greenhouse gas emissions through transportation. By growing your own food, you eliminate the need for transportation and reduce the overall carbon footprint of your meals.

• **Decreasing Packaging Waste**: Many store-bought fruits and vegetables come wrapped in plastic packaging, which ends up in landfills. Growing your own food means you can harvest it without the need for packaging, reducing plastic waste.

• **Lowering Water Use**: Growing food at home allows you to take control of water use. You can implement water-efficient methods like rainwater harvesting or drip irrigation to ensure that your plants get the right amount of water, without the waste.

2. Health Benefits:

• **Access to Fresh, Chemical-Free Produce**: Home gardens allow you to grow your food without pesticides or synthetic fertilizers, meaning you can enjoy healthier, chemical-free produce.

• **Physical and Mental Well-Being**: Gardening is a form of exercise that promotes physical activity and mental well-being. It provides a sense of accomplishment and connection to nature, which can help reduce stress and improve overall health.

3. Cost Savings:

• **Saving Money**: Growing your own food, especially herbs, vegetables, and fruits, can reduce your grocery bill. Once your garden is established, the cost of seeds, water, and occasional supplies is minimal compared to buying fresh produce at the store.

By dedicating space to a home garden, you can actively participate in sustainable living while reaping the personal and environmental benefits.

Native Plants and Organic Gardening: Supporting Biodiversity and Reducing Chemical Use

Native plants and organic gardening practices not only create beautiful, low-maintenance landscapes but also help protect and support local ecosystems. By focusing on plant species that are naturally adapted to your region, you can reduce the need for water, pesticides, and fertilizers while promoting biodiversity.

1. Native Plants:

• **Supporting Local Wildlife**: Native plants provide food and habitat for local pollinators, birds, insects, and other wildlife. Many of these plants have evolved alongside local wildlife, making them a vital part of the ecosystem.

• **Lower Maintenance and Water Needs**: Native plants are adapted to the local climate, so they require less water, fewer fertilizers, and less care compared to non-native species. This makes them ideal for sustainable landscaping, as they thrive with minimal intervention.

• **Invasive Species Prevention**: Non-native plants can sometimes become invasive, outcompeting native species and disrupting local ecosystems. By choosing native plants, you help maintain the balance of local habitats.

2. Organic Gardening:

• **Reducing Chemical Use**: Organic gardening avoids the use of synthetic pesticides, herbicides, and fertilizers. Instead, it relies on natural methods, such as composting, crop rotation, and companion planting, to promote plant health and pest control.

• **Soil Health**: Organic gardening practices enrich the soil with organic matter, fostering a healthy, thriving ecosystem for your plants. Healthy soil holds more water and nutrients, which reduces the need for chemical fertilizers and helps create a more resilient garden.

• **Pollution Reduction**: By avoiding chemical pesticides and fertilizers, organic gardening helps protect local water sources from contamination, as chemicals can run off into nearby streams and rivers, polluting aquatic ecosystems.

Planting native species and practicing organic gardening are key strategies for creating a sustainable garden that supports biodiversity and reduces your environmental impact.

Water-Efficient Landscaping: Designing Your Garden to Minimize Water Waste

Water is a precious resource, and sustainable landscaping focuses on designing gardens that require minimal water. By using water-efficient techniques, you can reduce your water usage while maintaining a beautiful, functional garden.

1. Drought-Tolerant Plants:

• **Choosing Water-Efficient Plants**: Many plants are drought-tolerant and can survive with little water once established. These plants, often referred to as "xeriscaping" plants, are well-suited to dry climates and can thrive with minimal watering. Examples include succulents, lavender, and native grasses.

• **Grouping Plants by Water Needs**: When designing your garden, group plants with similar water needs together. This allows you to water efficiently and avoid over-watering plants that require less moisture.

2. Irrigation Systems:

• **Drip Irrigation**: A drip irrigation system delivers water directly to the plant roots, minimizing water waste through evaporation or runoff. It is an efficient way to water your garden, especially during dry spells.

• **Soaker Hoses**: These hoses allow water to seep out slowly, ensuring that water reaches the plant roots rather than running off the surface. Soaker hoses are ideal for vegetable gardens and flower beds.

• **Rainwater Harvesting**: Collecting rainwater in barrels or storage tanks is a sustainable way to water your garden. Rainwater is naturally soft and free from chemicals, making it ideal for plants. Setting up a rainwater harvesting system can significantly reduce your reliance on municipal water sources.

3. Mulching:

• **Retaining Moisture**: Mulch is a layer of organic or inorganic material placed around plants to help retain soil moisture. It also helps suppress weeds and regulate soil temperature.

• **Organic Mulch**: Organic mulches, like straw, wood chips, or leaves, break down over time, enriching the soil and providing additional nutrients to your plants.

By incorporating these water-efficient techniques into your landscaping, you can reduce water waste and create a garden that is both beautiful and sustainable.

Composting: Creating Nutrient-Rich Soil and Reducing Food Scraps

Composting is a natural process that turns organic waste into nutrient-rich soil, reducing the need for chemical fertilizers and reducing the amount of food waste that ends up in landfills.

Composting is an essential practice for sustainable gardening and can significantly improve the health of your garden.

1. The Basics of Composting:

• **What to Compost**: Kitchen scraps like vegetable peels, coffee grounds, and fruit scraps, along with yard waste like grass clippings, leaves, and plant trimmings, can all be composted. Avoid adding meat, dairy, or oily foods, as these can attract pests.

• **Composting Methods**: There are several ways to compost, including using a compost bin, pile, or vermiculture (worm composting). Choose a method that fits your space and lifestyle.

• **The Composting Process**: Composting requires a balance of green (nitrogen-rich) and brown (carbon-rich) materials. Green materials include food scraps and grass clippings, while brown materials include leaves, straw, and cardboard. The compost needs air (oxygen) and moisture to decompose properly, so be sure to turn the pile regularly to keep it aerated.

2. Benefits of Composting:

• **Reducing Waste**: Composting helps divert food scraps and yard waste from landfills, where they would otherwise produce harmful methane gas as they decompose.

• **Improving Soil Health**: The compost created is rich in organic matter, which improves soil structure, water retention, and fertility. Healthy soil leads to stronger plants and reduced need for chemical fertilizers.

• **Sustainable Fertilizer**: Instead of purchasing synthetic fertilizers, compost provides a natural, eco-friendly alternative that nourishes your plants.

Composting is a simple, effective way to reduce waste, improve your garden's soil, and contribute to a more sustainable lifestyle.

To Keep In Mind: Sustainable gardening and landscaping practices, such as growing your own food, planting native species, conserving water, and composting, can significantly reduce your environmental footprint while creating a beautiful and functional outdoor space. By embracing these practices, you can support local ecosystems, improve soil health, conserve resources, and reduce waste. Whether you're starting a small herb garden or redesigning your entire landscape, every step toward sustainable gardening helps create a greener, more resilient planet.

40 mini

Chapter 10
Eco-Friendly Home Improvements

Home improvements offer a significant opportunity to reduce your environmental footprint and increase energy efficiency. Whether you're renovating an existing space or building from scratch, incorporating sustainable practices and eco-friendly materials can help you create a healthier, more energy-efficient home. In this chapter, we'll explore sustainable building materials, green certifications, how to reduce the carbon footprint of your home, and the innovative concept of green roofs and walls.

Sustainable Building Materials: What to Consider When Renovating or Building a Home

Sustainable building materials are those that have minimal environmental impact during their production, use, and disposal. Choosing these materials is crucial for reducing your home's carbon footprint and contributing to a greener planet.

1. Types of Sustainable Materials:

• **Recycled Materials**: Using recycled materials such as reclaimed wood, steel, or glass helps divert waste from landfills and reduces the need for new raw materials. Recycled content reduces energy consumption and lowers environmental impact.

• **Bamboo**: Bamboo is a rapidly renewable material that grows much faster than traditional hardwoods, making it an excellent choice for flooring, cabinetry, and furniture. It is durable, versatile, and has a low environmental impact.

• **Recycled Steel**: Steel is one of the most recycled materials in the world. Using recycled steel in construction reduces the need for mining, lowers energy usage, and helps keep valuable materials out of landfills.

• **Hempcrete**: Made from hemp stalks, lime, and water, hempcrete is a sustainable alternative to concrete. It is lightweight, energy-efficient, and carbon-negative, as it absorbs CO_2 during its growth process.

• **Cork**: Cork is a renewable, biodegradable material that can be used for flooring, insulation, and wall coverings. It's harvested without damaging the tree, making it a sustainable choice for the home.

• **Low-VOC Paints and Finishes**: Volatile organic compounds (VOCs) in paints and finishes contribute to indoor air pollution. Low-VOC or VOC-free paints and finishes reduce harmful emissions, improving air quality and creating a healthier living environment.

2. Other Considerations:

• **Locally Sourced Materials**: Sourcing materials locally reduces the carbon footprint associated with transportation, supports local economies, and ensures the use of materials suited to your region's climate.

• **Durability**: Choosing durable materials that will last for many years helps reduce the frequency of replacements, minimizing waste and the need for new resources.

• **Energy Efficiency**: Select materials that contribute to the home's energy efficiency, such as insulating materials that help maintain a comfortable indoor temperature with minimal energy use.

By using sustainable building materials, you not only reduce your environmental impact but also create a healthier, more energy-efficient home.

Green Certifications: Understanding Eco-Certifications Like LEED and Energy Star

Green certifications are third-party verifications that ensure a building meets specific environmental and energy-efficiency standards. These certifications help homeowners and builders choose products and designs that align with sustainable building practices.

1. LEED (Leadership in Energy and Environmental Design):

• **What It Is**: LEED is one of the most recognized and respected green building certification programs in the world. It evaluates buildings based on energy efficiency, water conservation, sustainable materials, indoor air quality, and more.

• **How It Works**: LEED certification is awarded in different levels (Certified, Silver, Gold, and Platinum) based on points earned in various categories, such as sustainable site development, water efficiency, energy use, and innovation in design.

• **Why It's Important**: A LEED-certified home is designed to use resources more efficiently, reduce waste, and improve the health and well-being of its inhabitants. It's an investment that can lead to long-term savings on utilities while minimizing environmental impact.

2. Energy Star:

• **What It Is**: The Energy Star program is a government-backed certification that helps homeowners identify energy-efficient appliances, building materials, and systems. Products that meet Energy Star standards use less energy, reduce greenhouse gas emissions, and save money on utility bills.

• **How It Works**: Energy Star evaluates products such as appliances, windows, insulation, and lighting to ensure they meet high energy efficiency standards. Homes with Energy Star certifications are built or renovated to use energy more efficiently, keeping energy consumption low while maintaining comfort.

• **Why It's Important**: Choosing Energy Star-certified products helps reduce your home's carbon footprint, lowers energy bills, and ensures your home operates with minimal environmental impact.

3. Other Certifications to Consider:

• **Passive House (Passivhaus)**: Passive House is a certification focused on ultra-low energy buildings that require little to no heating or cooling. This certification ensures that the home is airtight, well-insulated, and energy-efficient, creating a comfortable indoor environment while minimizing energy use.

• **Living Building Challenge**: The Living Building Challenge is one of the most rigorous environmental certifications, focusing on sustainability, social equity, and regenerative design. Buildings that achieve this certification must meet a series of stringent performance standards related to energy, water, materials, and indoor air quality.

By opting for green-certified materials and systems, you can ensure that your home meets high sustainability standards and contributes to a healthier planet.

Reducing the Carbon Footprint of Your Home: How to Make Your Home More Energy-Efficient

Making your home more energy-efficient is one of the most effective ways to reduce its carbon footprint. By using less energy, you can lower your utility bills and reduce greenhouse gas emissions. Here are some practical ways to improve your home's energy efficiency:

1. Insulation and Sealing:

• **Insulate Your Home**: Proper insulation keeps your home warm in the winter and cool in the summer, reducing the need for heating and air conditioning. Common areas to insulate include the attic, walls, floors, and windows.

• **Seal Gaps and Leaks**: Check for drafts around windows, doors, and vents. Sealing these gaps with weatherstripping or caulk helps prevent heat loss and keeps your home comfortable.

2. Energy-Efficient Appliances:

• **Upgrade to Energy-Efficient Appliances**: When replacing appliances, choose those with the Energy Star label, which indicates they meet high energy efficiency standards. Energy-efficient appliances, such as refrigerators, washing machines, and dishwashers, use less energy, saving you money and reducing your home's carbon footprint.

• **Smart Thermostats**: A smart thermostat learns your heating and cooling preferences and adjusts temperatures automatically to maximize energy savings. These thermostats can be programmed to optimize your home's energy use, reducing heating and cooling costs.

3. Renewable Energy:

• **Solar Power**: Installing solar panels is an excellent way to reduce your home's reliance on fossil fuels. Solar energy is renewable, abundant, and can significantly reduce your electricity bills.

• **Wind Power**: If you live in a suitable location, small wind turbines can generate renewable energy for your home.

• **Geothermal Heating and Cooling**: Geothermal systems use the stable temperature of the earth to heat and cool your home. They are highly efficient and can significantly reduce energy use.

4. Lighting:

• **Switch to LED Bulbs**: LED bulbs use far less energy than incandescent bulbs and last longer. Switching to LED lighting throughout your home can significantly reduce your electricity consumption.

• **Use Natural Light**: Maximize natural light by strategically placing windows, skylights, and light-colored walls that reflect sunlight into your home. This reduces the need for artificial lighting during the day.

By focusing on energy efficiency, you can create a comfortable and eco-friendly home that minimizes its carbon footprint.

Green Roofs and Walls: How Incorporating Plants

Into Your Home Design Can Improve Energy Efficiency

Green roofs and walls are innovative, sustainable design features that can enhance energy efficiency while promoting biodiversity. These green installations involve planting vegetation on rooftops or building walls, offering both aesthetic and environmental benefits.

1. Green Roofs:

• **What They Are**: A green roof involves covering the roof of a building with vegetation, typically planted in a layer of soil or growing medium. Green roofs help insulate buildings, reduce the urban heat island effect, and improve stormwater management.

• **Energy Efficiency**: Green roofs provide natural insulation, reducing the need for air conditioning in the summer and heating in the winter. They help regulate indoor temperatures, reducing energy consumption.

• **Biodiversity and Stormwater Management**: Green roofs create habitats for birds and insects, support local biodiversity, and absorb rainwater, preventing runoff and reducing the strain on stormwater systems.

2. Green Walls (Living Walls):

• **What They Are**: Green walls, also known as living walls, are vertical gardens that are installed on the exterior or interior of a building. These walls use a modular system that allows plants to grow vertically, creating a green façade that provides both aesthetic and environmental benefits.

• **Energy Efficiency**: Green walls help insulate buildings, reducing the need for heating and cooling. They act as natural air conditioners by reducing heat absorption and providing shade.

• **Air Quality Improvement**: Green walls can also improve indoor air quality by filtering pollutants and releasing oxygen.

By incorporating green roofs and walls into your home design, you can enhance energy efficiency, promote biodiversity, and contribute to a more sustainable urban environment.

To Keep In Mind: Eco-friendly home improvements—such as using sustainable materials, obtaining green certifications, improving energy efficiency, and incorporating green roofs and walls—can significantly reduce your home's environmental impact. These improvements not only save you money on utilities but also contribute to a healthier, more sustainable world. Whether you're renovating an existing space or building from scratch, embracing eco-friendly design choices will create a comfortable, energy-efficient home that reflects your commitment to sustainability.

Chapter 11
Sustainable Personal Care and Health

Personal care and health products are essential in our daily lives, but many of these items come with hidden environmental costs. From plastic packaging to chemicals that harm ecosystems, the personal care industry can have a significant impact on the planet. However, by making conscious choices, we can align our self-care routines with sustainable practices that not only benefit our health but also the environment. In this chapter, we'll explore how to choose eco-friendly beauty products, incorporate natural alternatives, and make sustainable choices in health and hygiene. We'll also discuss the important connection between personal health and environmental well-being.

Eco-Friendly Beauty Products: What to Look for in Skincare and Makeup Products

As consumers become more aware of the environmental impact of beauty products, many are turning to eco-friendly alternatives. When selecting beauty products, it's important to prioritize those that are not only safe for your skin but also kind to the planet.

1. Ingredients to Look For:

• **Natural and Organic Ingredients**: Choose beauty products made with natural and organic ingredients that are free from harsh chemicals, parabens, and synthetic fragrances. Organic products are grown without the use of pesticides or chemical fertilizers, making them gentler on the environment and your skin.

• **Vegan and Cruelty-Free**: Vegan beauty products are made without any animal-derived ingredients, and cruelty-free products are not tested on animals. These options promote ethical beauty standards and support animal rights.

• **Plant-Based Oils**: Look for plant-based oils such as argan oil, coconut oil, or jojoba oil, which are sustainably sourced and gentle on the skin. These oils provide moisture and nourishment without harmful additives.

• **Non-Toxic Formulas**: Avoid beauty products containing harmful ingredients like phthalates, sulfates, and formaldehyde, which can be damaging to both your health and the environment.

2. Packaging:

• **Minimal and Recyclable Packaging**: Opt for products that use minimal or recyclable packaging. Glass containers and metal tins are more sustainable options compared to plastic bottles. Look for brands that prioritize packaging made from recycled or biodegradable materials.

• **Refillable Packaging**: Some beauty brands offer refillable containers, which help reduce waste and the need for single-use packaging. This can significantly cut down on plastic waste and is a more sustainable choice for frequent beauty product users.

3. Eco-Friendly Beauty Brands:

• Many beauty brands now focus on sustainability by using natural ingredients, eco-friendly packaging, and cruelty-free practices.

Some brands even offer environmentally friendly alternatives for makeup removers, shampoos, and lotions, allowing you to swap out traditional products for greener options.

By choosing eco-friendly beauty products, you can minimize the environmental impact of your beauty routine while supporting companies that prioritize sustainability.

Natural Alternatives: How to Replace Chemical-Laden Products with Natural Solutions

Many conventional beauty and personal care products contain chemicals that can be harmful to both your body and the environment. Fortunately, there are natural alternatives available that can help reduce exposure to toxic substances while promoting healthier skin and hair.

1. Natural Skincare:

• **DIY Face Masks and Scrubs**: You can create your own skincare products using ingredients from your kitchen. For example, honey and oatmeal can be used as gentle exfoliants, while avocado and yogurt can be used to make hydrating face masks.

• **Aloe Vera and Coconut Oil**: Both aloe vera and coconut oil are popular natural moisturizers that are gentle on the skin and have numerous benefits. Aloe vera has soothing properties, while coconut oil is an excellent hydrating and anti-inflammatory agent.

• **Essential Oils**: Essential oils such as lavender, tea tree, and eucalyptus can be used in your skincare routine to promote healing, balance skin tone, and reduce inflammation. They're also effective in replacing artificial fragrances in personal care products.

2. Natural Hair Care:

• **Shampoo Bars and Natural Shampoos**: Traditional liquid shampoos often come in plastic bottles and contain harsh chemicals. Instead, try shampoo bars made from natural ingredients like shea butter, coconut oil, and essential oils. These bars are often plastic-free and more eco-friendly.

• **Apple Cider Vinegar Rinse**: Instead of chemical-laden conditioners, use a diluted apple cider vinegar rinse to balance your hair's pH and add shine. It's a simple, natural solution that helps remove buildup and improve hair health.

• **DIY Hair Masks**: You can create nourishing hair masks using ingredients such as honey, olive oil, and avocado. These provide natural hydration and can help with various hair issues like dryness and frizz.

3. Natural Oral Care:

• **Baking Soda and Essential Oils**: Baking soda is a natural alternative to toothpaste and can help whiten teeth and freshen breath. Adding a few drops of peppermint or tea tree essential oil can enhance its cleansing properties.

• **Natural Toothbrushes**: Choose toothbrushes with bamboo handles, which are biodegradable and compostable, instead of plastic ones. Some brands offer bamboo toothbrushes with recyclable bristles or natural, eco-friendly toothpaste options.

Switching to natural alternatives allows you to avoid harmful chemicals and reduce your environmental footprint while maintaining your personal care routine.

Eco-Friendly Health and Hygiene: Sustainable Alternatives for Toothbrushes, Razors, and More

In addition to beauty products, everyday health and hygiene items also contribute to waste and environmental harm. Fortunately, there are many eco-friendly alternatives that can help reduce the impact of personal care products.

1. Toothbrushes:

• **Bamboo Toothbrushes**: Bamboo toothbrushes are biodegradable and compostable, unlike their plastic counterparts, which can take hundreds of years to break down. Bamboo is a renewable resource, making it a sustainable option for oral care.

• **Toothpaste Tablets or Powder**: Traditional toothpaste tubes often contain plastic and are difficult to recycle. Toothpaste tablets or powders come in recyclable glass containers or compostable packaging, providing a sustainable alternative to tube-based toothpaste.

2. Razors:

• **Safety Razors**: Traditional disposable razors often have plastic handles and cannot be recycled. Safety razors, on the other hand, have metal handles that can be reused indefinitely. The razor blades are also recyclable, making them a more sustainable option for shaving.

• **Shaving Brushes and Soaps**: Instead of using shaving gels that come in plastic cans, use natural shaving soaps and brushes. These products are often sold in eco-friendly packaging, reducing waste and promoting a more sustainable shaving routine.

3. Period Products:

• **Menstrual Cups and Reusable Pads**: Disposable period products such as tampons and pads contribute significantly to waste. Menstrual cups and reusable cloth pads are more sustainable alternatives that can be used for years, reducing the need for single-use products.

• **Organic Cotton Products**: If you prefer disposable products, look for those made with organic cotton, which is grown without harmful pesticides and synthetic fertilizers. These products are biodegradable and gentler on the environment.

4. Eco-Friendly Deodorants:

• **Plastic-Free Deodorants**: Many conventional deodorants come in plastic packaging, but there are now eco-friendly options that come in compostable or recyclable containers. Look for deodorants that use natural ingredients, such as baking soda, coconut oil, and essential oils, instead of synthetic chemicals.

By replacing everyday hygiene products with eco-friendly alternatives, you can reduce plastic waste and avoid harmful chemicals while maintaining good health and personal hygiene.

Holistic Health and Sustainability: The Connection Between Personal Health and Environmental Well-Being

Personal health and environmental sustainability are deeply interconnected. What's good for your body is often good for the planet, and vice versa. A holistic approach to health that incorporates sustainable practices benefits both your well-being and the environment.

1. The Impact of Chemicals on Health and the Environment:

• Many conventional beauty and personal care products contain harmful chemicals that can have negative effects on both your health and the environment. Pesticides, phthalates, and parabens can contribute to health issues such as hormone disruption, skin irritation, and allergies. Additionally, when these chemicals enter water systems through washing or disposal, they can harm aquatic life and pollute ecosystems.

• By choosing natural, organic products that avoid harmful chemicals, you are not only protecting your body from potential toxins but also helping to preserve the environment from chemical contamination.

2. Sustainable Diet and Health:

• The food you eat plays a significant role in both your personal health and the health of the planet. A diet focused on plant-based foods, whole grains, and organic produce can improve your health while reducing your carbon footprint. Sustainable food choices often involve less resource-intensive production methods and contribute to reducing the environmental impact of agriculture.

• A healthy lifestyle that includes exercise, a balanced diet, and mindfulness practices not only improves your well-being but also reduces your overall environmental impact by promoting sustainable food choices and a connection to the natural world.

3. Mind-Body Connection:

• Embracing sustainable personal care products, a clean and non-toxic environment, and holistic health practices encourages a deeper connection to the planet and its ecosystems. This awareness fosters a sense of responsibility to protect the environment, leading to more eco-conscious choices in all areas of life.

• A sustainable lifestyle that nurtures both your physical health and environmental well-being creates a positive feedback loop, where each contributes to the other, resulting in a healthier you and a healthier planet.

By adopting a holistic approach to health that incorporates sustainability, you can create a lifestyle that supports both personal well-being and environmental preservation.

To Keep In Mind: Sustainable personal care and health choices are an important aspect of living a greener, more mindful life. By opting for eco-friendly beauty products, natural alternatives, and sustainable hygiene products, you can reduce your environmental impact while promoting personal health. The connection between health and the environment is undeniable, and making conscious choices in your personal care routine contributes to the broader goal of a

Chapter 12
Green Office Practices

In today's world, sustainability extends beyond the home and into the workplace. Whether you're working in a traditional office setting or from home, adopting eco-friendly practices at work can make a significant impact on reducing your carbon footprint and promoting a sustainable environment. This chapter will guide you through practical steps to make your office more eco-friendly by choosing sustainable office supplies, reducing energy consumption, and minimizing waste. We'll also discuss how remote work can play a role in sustainability and how to create a waste-free office.

Eco-Friendly Office Supplies: How to Choose Sustainable Stationery and Equipment

The items you use daily in the office — from pens and paper to computers and printers — can contribute to a significant environmental footprint. Switching to eco-friendly office supplies is one of the easiest ways to minimize your impact and promote sustainability at work.

1. Sustainable Paper Products:

• **Recycled Paper**: Instead of using virgin paper, choose paper products made from post-consumer recycled content. Look for paper with a high percentage of recycled material and ensure it's certified by standards like the Forest Stewardship Council (FSC), which ensures responsible forest management.

• **Tree-Free Paper**: Consider using paper alternatives made from bamboo, hemp, or other sustainable fibers. These materials require less water, energy, and pesticides to produce than traditional wood-pulp paper.

• **Digital Note-Taking**: Opt for digital notes and avoid printing whenever possible. Use tablets, computers, or digital apps to take notes and keep records, reducing paper waste.

2. Eco-Friendly Stationery:

• **Non-Toxic and Recycled Pens**: Choose pens and markers made from recycled plastic or materials like bamboo. Avoid disposable pens, which contribute to plastic waste. Consider refillable pens, which can be used for years.

• **Sustainable Notebooks**: Look for notebooks made from recycled paper or plant-based materials like sugarcane, which use fewer resources and have a lower environmental impact. Some brands also offer notebooks that are fully biodegradable.

• **Eco-Conscious Desk Organizers**: Choose office organizers made from sustainable materials such as bamboo, recycled plastic, or upcycled wood. These materials are not only eco-friendly but often more durable than conventional plastic products.

3. Energy-Efficient Office Equipment:

• **Energy-Efficient Electronics**: When purchasing office equipment like computers, monitors, and printers, look for

ENERGY STAR-rated products, which are designed to consume less energy. Additionally, opt for refurbished electronics to reduce the environmental impact of manufacturing new devices.

• **Eco-Friendly Printers and Cartridges**: If printing is necessary, use energy-efficient printers and refillable ink or toner cartridges. Avoid disposable plastic cartridges and opt for recycled or refillable alternatives. Reducing the frequency of printing also cuts down on paper waste.

• **Paperless Workflow**: Digitize documents and utilize cloud storage services to keep your files organized and accessible without the need for physical copies. Tools like electronic signatures and digital note-taking apps help reduce dependency on paper.

Energy Efficiency in the Workplace: Reducing Energy Use in the Office Environment

Energy consumption in the workplace can have a significant environmental impact, especially if the office relies heavily on electricity for lighting, heating, and powering electronic devices. By adopting energy-efficient practices, businesses and individuals can reduce their energy use and lower their carbon footprint.

1. Efficient Lighting:

• **LED Lighting**: Switch out traditional incandescent or fluorescent bulbs for LED lighting, which uses significantly less energy and lasts longer. In addition to energy savings, LED lights emit less heat, which can help with cooling costs in the office.

• **Motion-Sensor Lights**: Install motion-sensor lighting in less frequently used spaces such as bathrooms, hallways, and conference rooms. These lights automatically turn off when no one is present, reducing unnecessary energy consumption.

• **Natural Lighting**: Maximize natural light by opening blinds and arranging your workspace near windows. Natural lighting is not only better for your well-being but also reduces the need for artificial lighting during the day.

2. Energy-Efficient Office Appliances:

• **Smart Thermostats**: Install a smart thermostat in the office to optimize heating and cooling. A programmable thermostat can help reduce energy use by adjusting temperatures based on office occupancy and time of day.

• **Energy-Efficient HVAC Systems**: Ensure that your heating, ventilation, and air conditioning (HVAC) system is energy-efficient and well-maintained. Regular maintenance, such as cleaning filters and ensuring proper insulation, can reduce energy consumption and improve the system's efficiency.

• **Power Strips and Energy-Saving Mode**: Encourage employees to turn off their computers, monitors, and other devices when not in use. Use power strips to easily disconnect devices and prevent "phantom" energy consumption when equipment is left on standby mode.

3. Remote Work and Hybrid Office Models:

• With the rise of remote work, many employees no longer need to commute to a physical office every day. This reduces energy consumption in office buildings and lowers carbon emissions from transportation. Encourage employees to work from home or adopt a hybrid work model where they spend fewer days in the office, thereby contributing to overall energy savings.

Remote Work and Sustainability: How Working From Home Can Reduce Your Carbon Footprint

Remote work offers a unique opportunity to reduce both energy consumption and transportation-related emissions. By eliminating the daily commute, employees can cut down on their carbon footprint significantly. In this section, we'll explore how working from home can benefit the environment and how you can ensure that your home office is sustainable.

1. Reduced Commute:

• **Lower Carbon Emissions**: One of the most significant environmental benefits of remote work is the reduction in emissions from commuting. A single round-trip commute by car can result in several kilograms of carbon dioxide (CO_2) emissions. With remote work, employees eliminate the need for daily car trips, leading to fewer emissions and a cleaner environment.

• **Reduced Traffic Congestion**: Fewer people on the roads mean less traffic congestion, which not only reduces carbon emissions but also helps cut down on air pollution and noise.

2. Efficient Home Office Practices:

• **Energy-Efficient Appliances**: In your home office, use energy-efficient devices such as laptops (which consume less energy than desktop computers) and LED lighting. Unplug devices when they're not in use to prevent wasting energy.

• **Sustainable Office Furniture**: Choose furniture made from sustainable materials, such as recycled metal or wood sourced from certified sustainable forests. Repurpose or upcycle old furniture to avoid the environmental cost of manufacturing new items.

• **Eco-Friendly Home Office Supplies**: Use recycled paper, natural cleaning products, and non-toxic supplies in your home office. When purchasing new office equipment or supplies, prioritize eco-friendly brands that are committed to sustainability.

3. Mental Health and Sustainability:

• Working from home can also contribute to mental well-being, which indirectly supports environmental sustainability. Employees who work from home tend to experience less stress related to commuting and have more flexibility, leading to a better work-life balance and overall healthier lifestyles. A healthier workforce is more likely to be environmentally conscious and motivated to adopt sustainable practices.

Waste-Free Office: Tips for Creating a Paperless, Plastic-Free Office

In addition to reducing energy consumption, creating a waste-free office is essential to promoting sustainability. Paper and plastic waste can accumulate quickly in an office environment, but with a few simple changes, you can drastically reduce your environmental impact.

1. Going Paperless:

• **Digital Documentation**: Encourage employees to digitize all documents and use cloud-based systems for file storage. Electronic documents can be accessed, shared, and edited without ever needing to print.

• **Paperless Communication**: Rely on digital communication tools such as email, instant messaging, and video calls instead of using paper memos, letters, or faxes. Use shared calendars, virtual meetings, and collaborative workspaces to minimize paper use.

• **Recycle Paper**: For any paper that does need to be used, ensure that it's recycled properly. Place recycling bins throughout the office and ensure that employees are aware of the importance of recycling.

2. Reducing Plastic Use:

• **Reusable Containers**: Eliminate single-use plastics by encouraging the use of reusable containers, water bottles, and coffee mugs. Offer employees reusable lunch containers and utensils to reduce plastic waste from disposable packaging.

• **Plastic-Free Office Events**: When hosting meetings or events, avoid plastic cups, plates, and utensils. Instead, use reusable or compostable alternatives. Provide employees with eco-friendly options for snacks, drinks, and catering.

• **Plastic-Free Stationery**: As mentioned earlier, choose eco-friendly stationery and office supplies made from recycled or biodegradable materials. Avoid plastic pens, binders, and other office items made from non-sustainable plastic.

To Keep In Mind: Adopting green office practices not only contributes to sustainability but can also improve the efficiency and productivity of your workplace. By switching to eco-friendly office supplies, reducing energy consumption, and minimizing waste, you can create a work environment that is both environmentally responsible and cost-effective. Whether you work in a traditional office or from home, making green changes in the workplace can have a positive and lasting impact on the planet.

Chapter 13
Green Travel and Eco-Friendly Vacations

Traveling can be an incredible way to explore new places, cultures, and experiences, but it also has an environmental impact. The carbon footprint of transportation, waste generated during travel, and the energy used in accommodations can contribute to environmental degradation. However, there are many ways to make your travel more sustainable and minimize its negative impact on the planet. This chapter will guide you on how to choose eco-friendly destinations, pack with sustainability in mind, find eco-conscious accommodations, and adopt green travel habits.

Choosing Eco-Friendly Destinations: How to Support Sustainable Tourism

When planning your next vacation, consider how the destination supports sustainable tourism practices. By choosing destinations that prioritize conservation, responsible tourism, and community support, you can ensure that your travels have a positive impact on the environment and local communities.

1. Sustainable Tourism Practices:

• **Eco-Certified Destinations**: Look for destinations that are recognized for their commitment to sustainability. Many destinations around the world have earned eco-certifications, such as Green Key or EarthCheck, which indicate that they follow sustainable tourism practices. These destinations focus on preserving natural resources, supporting local economies, and minimizing their environmental impact.

• **Supporting Local Communities**: Choose destinations that emphasize community-driven tourism. Spend money in local businesses, buy locally made crafts, and engage in activities that support cultural preservation. Tourism can provide a vital source of income for local communities, so supporting businesses that are committed to responsible tourism can help maintain the region's cultural and environmental integrity.

• **Nature Conservation**: Opt for destinations that actively protect their natural environment, such as national parks or wildlife sanctuaries. These areas often have strong conservation efforts in place to protect ecosystems and endangered species, ensuring that future generations can also enjoy the beauty of these places.

2. Offsetting Carbon Emissions:

• **Carbon Offset Programs**: If you must travel by plane or other high-emission transportation methods, consider purchasing carbon offsets. Many airlines and travel agencies offer the option to offset the emissions generated by your flight. This typically involves contributing to projects such as reforestation, renewable energy, or methane capture, which help balance out your travel-related emissions.

Packing Light: How Packing Less Reduces Your Environmental Impact

Packing light is not only a smart travel practice; it's also an eco-friendly one. The more you pack, the heavier your luggage, which can result in more fuel being used for transportation. Additionally, packing light helps reduce the demand for overconsumption and waste.

1. Reducing the Carbon Footprint of Travel:

• **Lighter Luggage**: Airlines and other transportation companies use fuel based on weight. By packing less, you reduce the overall weight of the vehicle, helping to conserve energy and reduce emissions. For instance, a lighter suitcase on an airplane helps reduce the aircraft's fuel consumption.

• **Minimizing Plastic Waste**: Packing fewer items also helps to avoid the need for excessive packaging, such as single-use plastic bags, bottles, and containers. This helps reduce the amount of plastic waste generated during your trip.

2. Travel Essentials:

• **Multi-Use Items**: Pack versatile clothing and products that can be used in multiple situations. Choose items that can be worn for various occasions and activities to minimize the number of clothes you bring. Opt for reusable toiletries, such as refillable shampoo bottles and a bamboo toothbrush, instead of single-use plastic versions.

• **Zero-Waste Travel Kit**: Consider bringing a travel kit that includes reusable items like a water bottle, tote bag, cutlery, and straws. Having these with you will help you avoid disposable plastics while on the go, reducing waste significantly.

Eco-Conscious Accommodations: How to Choose Eco-Friendly Hotels and Resorts

Where you stay during your travels can have a big impact on the environment. Choosing eco-conscious accommodations can help you support businesses that prioritize sustainability and reduce the environmental footprint of your trip.

1. Eco-Certified Hotels:

• **Green Certifications**: Look for hotels, resorts, and lodges that have earned eco-certifications like Green Key, EarthCheck, or Green Globe. These certifications ensure that accommodations follow strict environmental standards, such as energy conservation, waste management, water efficiency, and supporting local ecosystems.

• **Energy and Water Efficiency**: Many eco-conscious hotels implement energy-saving measures, such as using LED lights, motion-sensor lighting, or solar power. Some accommodations also reduce water consumption by using low-flow showers and taps and implementing linen and towel reuse programs to reduce laundry-related water usage.

2. Sustainable Practices:

• **Zero-Waste Hotels**: Some eco-friendly hotels have adopted zero-waste policies, focusing on reducing their environmental footprint by minimizing waste sent to landfills. Look for accommodations that provide composting facilities, offer bulk toiletries, and reduce plastic packaging.

• **Locally Sourced Food**: Choose accommodations that serve food made from local, organic ingredients. Many eco-friendly hotels source their food from local farmers or maintain their own gardens, reducing the carbon footprint associated with transportation and providing fresh, seasonal dishes.

• **Community Involvement**: Look for hotels that engage in community-based projects. Many eco-friendly resorts partner with local communities, providing jobs, supporting local culture, and engaging in philanthropic efforts that benefit both guests and the local population.

Sustainable Travel Habits: Reducing Waste and Energy Use While Traveling

Once you've chosen your destination, packed your bags, and booked your eco-friendly accommodations, it's time to adopt sustainable habits during your travels. Small actions, such as reducing waste and conserving energy, can go a long way in minimizing your environmental impact.

1. Transportation:

• **Public Transportation and Biking**: Once you reach your destination, opt for public transportation, bikes, or walking instead of renting a car. These options are not only more eco-friendly but also give you a chance to experience the area more intimately. Many cities offer bike-sharing programs, making it easy to get around sustainably.

• **Eco-Friendly Tours**: When booking tours or activities, choose companies that prioritize sustainability. Look for eco-friendly operators who focus on wildlife conservation, respect local cultures, and avoid overexploiting natural resources.

2. Reducing Waste:

• **Pack Reusable Items**: Bring reusable water bottles, coffee cups, and bags to reduce the use of single-use plastics. Many airports, restaurants, and tourist attractions now offer refilling stations, so you can avoid purchasing bottled water and reduce your plastic consumption.

• **Proper Waste Disposal**: Be mindful of where you dispose of waste. Always separate recyclables, compostables, and trash, and follow local guidelines for proper waste disposal. If the area you're visiting does not have good recycling programs, try to minimize your waste and bring any recyclables back home.

• **Avoid Mass Tourism Attractions**: Avoid crowded tourist spots that might be causing significant environmental strain. Instead, explore less-visited areas or destinations with strong conservation programs in place. This helps alleviate pressure on local ecosystems while supporting more responsible tourism practices.

3. Sustainable Food Choices:

• **Eating Local**: Support local restaurants that source ingredients locally and prepare traditional, sustainable dishes. Eating locally reduces the carbon footprint associated with food transportation and helps sustain local food culture.

• **Vegan and Plant-Based Meals**: Consider adopting a plant-based diet while traveling. Plant-based meals typically have a lower environmental impact compared to meat-based dishes, requiring fewer resources like water and energy to produce.

To Keep In Mind: Traveling sustainably doesn't mean sacrificing the joy of exploring new places; instead, it's about making conscious choices that protect the environment and support the local communities you visit. By choosing eco-friendly destinations, packing light, selecting sustainable accommodations, and adopting green travel habits, you can significantly reduce your environmental impact while still enjoying your vacation. Travel with intention, and you can help preserve the beauty of the world for future generations to experience.

Chapter 14
Supporting Sustainable Brands and Businesses

As consumers, we have the power to drive positive change in the marketplace. By supporting sustainable brands and businesses, we can encourage more companies to prioritize ethical and eco-friendly practices. This chapter will guide you through how to make informed decisions when shopping, understand the power of your purchasing choices, and identify certifications that signal truly sustainable brands. Additionally, we'll explore ways to advocate for sustainability and encourage businesses to adopt more responsible practices.

Ethical Shopping: How to Support Businesses with Strong Environmental and Social Responsibility

Ethical shopping involves choosing products and brands that align with your values, particularly in terms of environmental and social responsibility. By prioritizing these companies, you help create demand for sustainability in the marketplace.

1. Consider the Whole Supply Chain:

• **Materials and Production**: Look for brands that use sustainable materials, such as organic cotton, recycled fabrics, or natural fibers. Companies that prioritize ethical sourcing and production practices often ensure that workers are paid fairly and work in safe conditions.

• **Fair Labor Practices**: Support businesses that uphold fair labor practices and ensure safe working conditions. Ethical brands are transparent about their supply chains, ensuring their products are not made through exploitative labor or under poor conditions.

• **Environmental Impact**: Prioritize brands that actively work to minimize their carbon footprint, use renewable energy sources, reduce waste, and utilize eco-friendly packaging. These companies may also focus on minimizing water consumption, reducing chemical use, and preserving biodiversity.

2. Supporting Local Businesses:

• Whenever possible, support small businesses and local artisans who may offer sustainable alternatives. Shopping locally reduces the environmental costs associated with long-distance transportation and often supports businesses that are directly invested in their community's well-being and sustainability.

3. Conscious Consumption:

• Instead of indulging in impulse buying or constantly seeking the latest trends, practice mindful consumption by purchasing only what you truly need. Choose high-quality products that will last longer, reducing the need for replacements and minimizing waste.

The Power of Your Dollar: Understanding How Consumer Choices Drive Industry Change

Every purchase you make is a vote for the kind of world you want to live in. The collective choices of consumers shape the marketplace, and sustainable purchasing decisions send a clear message to companies about the importance of ethical and eco-friendly practices.

1. Shifting Industry Standards:

• **Consumer Demand**: When more people choose eco-friendly products or support ethical businesses, it pushes industries to change. Many companies have already started adopting sustainable practices in response to consumer demand for environmentally friendly products, and this trend is expected to continue.

• **Supporting Innovation**: By purchasing products from sustainable brands, you support the development of new technologies and innovations that reduce environmental impact. For example, brands that use plant-based or biodegradable packaging often lead the way in creating alternatives to single-use plastics.

2. Influencing Corporate Responsibility:

• **Lobbying for Change**: As a consumer, you have the ability to influence corporate practices by voicing your concerns or praising companies for their sustainability efforts. Many companies are now paying attention to customer feedback and adjusting their business practices accordingly. This could include adopting more sustainable packaging, improving labor practices, or committing to carbon neutrality.

Certifications and Labels: How to Identify Truly Sustainable Brands

Navigating the world of sustainable products can be challenging, as many brands use buzzwords like "green," "eco-friendly," or "sustainable" without backing up their claims. Certifications and labels can help you identify companies that are genuinely committed to environmental and social responsibility.

1. Common Eco-Certifications:

• **Fair Trade**: This certification ensures that products have been produced under fair labor conditions, with fair wages for workers and support for local communities. Fair Trade certification also promotes environmentally sustainable practices.

• **B Corp Certification**: B Corps are companies that meet high standards of social and environmental performance, accountability, and transparency. These companies balance purpose and profit, ensuring that their operations benefit society and the planet.

• **Certified Organic**: Products labeled as "organic" have been produced without synthetic pesticides or fertilizers. This certification promotes sustainable farming practices and protects biodiversity and soil health.

• **Cradle to Cradle (C2C)**: This certification focuses on the circular economy, ensuring that products are designed for continuous reuse and are made from materials that can be safely returned to the environment or reused in other products.

• **Energy Star**: Products with the Energy Star label meet strict energy efficiency guidelines, helping consumers save energy and reduce greenhouse gas emissions.

2. Eco-Friendly Packaging Labels:

• **Plastic-Free**: Products labeled as "plastic-free" or "plastic neutral" help reduce the amount of plastic waste entering landfills and oceans. Look for alternatives like biodegradable packaging or packaging made from recycled materials.

• **Recyclable or Compostable**: Many products now feature labels that indicate they can be recycled or composted. By choosing these products, you help reduce waste and support the circular economy.

3. Trustworthy Certifications:

• It's important to research and verify certifications before purchasing. Unfortunately, some businesses may use misleading or unverified labels. Look for certifications from reputable organizations to ensure that brands are truly committed to sustainable practices.

Advocating for Sustainability: How to Encourage Businesses and Organizations to Adopt Sustainable Practices

As consumers, we also have the power to advocate for sustainability within the businesses and organizations we interact with. Encouraging companies to adopt more sustainable practices can create ripple effects that reach beyond your own purchases.

1. Speaking Up:

• **Provide Feedback**: Reach out to companies to let them know that sustainability matters to you. Praise companies that are making a positive impact and share your concerns with businesses that could improve. Many businesses listen to customer feedback and take it into account when making decisions.

• **Start Conversations**: Advocate for sustainability by initiating discussions with friends, family, and colleagues. When you promote green habits, you help build a community of like-minded individuals who can collectively drive change in their personal and professional lives.

2. Supporting Policies for Sustainability:

• **Encourage Corporate Responsibility**: Support policies that promote sustainability and demand better practices from companies. For example, encourage businesses to disclose their carbon emissions, adopt renewable energy sources, or commit to zero-waste goals. Many businesses are responsive to regulations and public pressure.

• **Advocacy Groups and Campaigns**: Join or support organizations and campaigns that push for sustainable practices in various industries, from fashion to food production. These groups often lobby for changes in policy, improve corporate transparency, and work to raise awareness about environmental issues.

3. Collaborating with Companies:

• **Sustainability Initiatives**: Encourage your employer, or the companies you work with, to adopt sustainable practices. This could include reducing energy consumption in the workplace, offering sustainable products, or committing to a sustainability certification program. Leading by example can inspire others to take similar actions.

• **Transparency**: Push companies to be more transparent about their supply chains, environmental impact, and sustainability goals. The more transparent a company is about its practices, the more likely it is to hold itself accountable and improve over time.

To Keep In Mind: Supporting sustainable brands and businesses is a powerful way to drive positive environmental and social change. By making informed choices about the products you purchase, understanding the power of your consumer dollar, and advocating for businesses to adopt more responsible practices, you can contribute to a greener, fairer world. Remember, every small change counts. The more people demand ethical and eco-friendly products, the more companies will be motivated to adopt sustainable practices, creating a ripple effect that benefits the planet and its people.

Chapter 15
Creating a Sustainable Future: Your Next Steps

Sustainability is not a one-time effort, but an ongoing journey. By taking personal action, engaging with your community, and advocating for policy changes, you can contribute to a greener future. This chapter will guide you in setting actionable sustainability goals, fostering change in your community, supporting meaningful policy reforms, and remaining committed to the road ahead.

Setting Goals for a Greener Future: How to Create Personal Sustainability Goals

To create a sustainable future, it's important to start with specific, measurable, and achievable goals. Personal sustainability goals help you stay focused, track progress, and make a tangible impact on the environment.

1. Identify Areas for Improvement:

• **Assess Your Current Habits**: Reflect on your lifestyle and identify areas where you can reduce your environmental impact. This could include energy use, waste generation, transportation, food consumption, and more.

• **Choose Areas of Focus**: Select one or two aspects of your life to prioritize. For example, if you want to reduce waste, your goal could be to reduce your single-use plastic consumption by 50% over the next year. Alternatively, you might set a goal to reduce your carbon footprint by using public transport or biking instead of driving.

2. Set Smart Goals:

• **Specific**: Be clear about what you want to achieve. Instead of saying "I want to be more sustainable," try "I will reduce my water consumption by 30% within six months."

• **Measurable**: Choose goals that can be tracked. For instance, "I will compost 80% of my food waste" is measurable and provides clear progress markers.

• **Achievable**: Ensure your goals are realistic given your resources and timeframe. Avoid overwhelming yourself with unrealistic expectations.

• **Relevant**: Make sure your goals align with your personal values and lifestyle. Focus on what matters most to you.

• **Time-Bound**: Set deadlines to hold yourself accountable. For example, "I will reduce my plastic use by 50% by the end of the year" provides a clear timeline for achieving the goal.

3. Monitor and Celebrate Progress:

• Regularly track your progress and celebrate small victories. Each positive change, no matter how small, brings you closer to your long-term sustainability goals.

• Adjust your goals as needed. Sustainability is a journey, and goals can evolve as you learn and grow.

Engaging Your Community: Encouraging Sustainability in Your Neighborhood, Workplace, and Beyond

Creating a sustainable future goes beyond individual actions—it requires collective efforts. Engaging with your community, workplace, and other groups can amplify your impact and create lasting change.

1. Get Involved Locally:

• **Start with Your Neighborhood**: Organize or participate in local sustainability initiatives, such as community clean-ups, recycling drives, or urban gardening projects. Form a group to discuss ways your community can reduce its environmental impact.

• **Support Local Initiatives**: Support local farmers' markets, eco-friendly businesses, or neighborhood composting programs. By encouraging others to do the same, you help create a culture of sustainability in your local area.

2. Promote Sustainability at Work:

• **Workplace Sustainability**: Advocate for green initiatives at your workplace, such as reducing energy use, providing recycling programs, offering sustainable products, or switching to digital records instead of paper. Engage your colleagues to raise awareness and promote sustainable habits in the office.

• **Green Certifications**: Encourage your employer to pursue environmental certifications or green building standards (e.g., LEED). This can boost the organization's sustainability credentials and contribute to overall energy and resource savings.

3. Educate and Inspire Others:

• Use your knowledge of sustainability to educate those around you. Lead by example and share tips on reducing waste, conserving energy, and supporting eco-friendly businesses.

• Start or join online communities or local groups focused on sustainability. The more people you inspire, the more widespread the change becomes.

Advocating for Policy Change: How to Support Environmental Policies at the Local, National, and Global Levels

Sustainability isn't just a personal responsibility—it's also about advocating for systemic change. Environmental policies can influence everything from clean energy incentives to pollution regulation and corporate responsibility.

1. Support Local Environmental Initiatives:

• **Get Involved in Local Politics**: Attend town meetings, engage with local politicians, and advocate for sustainability measures in your community. Push for policies such as waste reduction programs, increased green spaces, and renewable energy incentives.

• **Raise Awareness**: Use your voice to raise awareness about important local environmental issues, such as air quality, water conservation, and land use. Support local campaigns that advocate for stronger environmental protections.

2. Push for National and Global Policy Reforms:

• **Engage with National Policy**: Stay informed about national environmental policies and legislation. Support policies that promote clean energy, carbon emissions reduction, and sustainable agriculture. Contact your representatives and let them know you support sustainable policies.

• **Join Global Movements**: Support international environmental organizations and movements that advocate for global change. From the Paris Climate Agreement to UN Sustainable Development Goals, many global initiatives rely on citizen advocacy to drive government and corporate action.

3. Lobby for Corporate Accountability:

• **Hold Businesses Accountable**: Advocate for policies that require businesses to disclose their environmental impact, adopt sustainable practices, and reduce waste. Push for stronger regulations around pollution, waste management, and ethical sourcing.

• **Support Transparency**: Encourage governments and organizations to support laws that require transparency in supply chains, carbon emissions, and sustainability claims.

The Road Ahead: The Ongoing Journey to Living Sustainably and Contributing to a Healthier Planet

The journey toward sustainability is not a destination, but a continual process of learning, evolving, and adapting. As you move forward, it's important to stay motivated and committed to the bigger picture.

1. Keep Learning and Evolving:

• Stay informed about new sustainability practices, technologies, and policies. As the world changes, new solutions to environmental challenges will emerge.

• Be open to change and continue to refine your habits. Sustainable living is a lifelong journey, and there will always be new ways to reduce your impact.

2. Celebrate Success and Progress:

• Take time to reflect on how far you've come. Celebrate the steps you've taken to live more sustainably, whether it's reducing waste, lowering your carbon footprint, or supporting ethical businesses.

• Share your success stories with others to inspire them to take their own steps toward sustainability.

3. Encourage Future Generations:

• Teach sustainability practices to younger generations. Share your knowledge and encourage children, students, and young adults to take care of the planet. The more we empower the next generation, the more likely they are to continue advocating for a healthier world.

4. Stay Committed:

• Remember, living sustainably is not about perfection but progress. It's about continuously finding ways to improve and adapt. By staying committed to sustainability, you contribute to creating a healthier, more equitable planet for future generations.

To Keep In Mind: The path to a sustainable future begins with each individual's commitment to making positive, lasting change. By setting clear sustainability goals, engaging with your community, advocating for policy change, and remaining dedicated to ongoing improvement, you can make a difference. Sustainability is a collective effort, and your contributions—no matter how small—help create a ripple effect that will continue to transform the world for the better. Together, we can build a greener, healthier, and more sustainable future.